Healthcare Delivery in the Information Age

For further volumes:
http://www.springer.com/series/8783

Healthcare Delivery in the Information Age

Mark Belkin • Brian Corbitt
Nilmini Wickramasinghe

Strategic ICT Planning
in Pathology

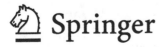 Springer

Mark Belkin
School of Business IT & Logistics
RMIT University
Melbourne, VIC
Australia

Brian Corbitt
School of Business IT & Logistics
RMIT University
Melbourne, VIC
Australia

Nilmini Wickramasinghe
Epworth HealthCare and RMIT University
Melbourne, VIC
Australia

ISBN 978-1-4899-9140-9   ISBN 978-1-4614-4478-7 (eBook)
DOI 10.1007/978-1-4614-4478-7
Springer New York Dordrecht Heidelberg London

Printed on acid-free paper

Springer is part of Springer Science+Business Media (www.springer.com)

*This series is dedicated to Leo Cussen:
learned scholar, colleague extraordinare
and good friend.*

Preface

In the current debates of healthcare economy, ICTs (Information Communication Technologies) continue to be heralded as the silver bullet (Wickramasinghe et al., IJBET 1:415–427, 2008). This should not come as a surprise, especially, since healthcare is an information rich, knowledge intensive environment. In order to treat and diagnose even a simple condition, a physician must combine many varied data elements and information (Wickramasinghe et al., Stud Health Technol Inform 137:147–162, 2008). Such multispectral data must be carefully integrated and synthesised to allow medically appropriate management of the disease (Wickramasinghe, IJIL 5: 201–216, 2008; Lubitz and Wickramasinghe, IJEH 4:415–428, 2006; Wickramasinghe et al., IJHTM 7: 303–318, 2006). Given the need to combine data and information into a coherent whole and then disseminate these findings to decision makers in a timely fashion, the benefits of ICT to support decision making of the physician and other actors throughout the healthcare system are clear (Wickramasinghe et al., IJHTM 7: 303–318, 2006; Wickramasinghe et al., Healthcare Knowledge Management Primer, Routledge, New York, 2006). In fact, we see the proliferation of many technologies such as EHR (electronic health records), PACS (picture archive computerized systems), CDSS (clinical decision support systems) etc. However and paradoxically, the more investment in ICT by healthcare the more global healthcare appears to be hampered by information chaos which in turn leads to inferior decision making, ineffective and inefficient operations, exponentially increasing costs and even loss of life (Wickramasinghe et al., Healthcare Knowledge Management Primer, Routledge, New York, 2006).

To date, one area that appears to have had little attention is the area of ICT use with regard to laboratory operations and pathology practices. This book serves to address this apparent void in the literature by providing an in-depth examination of the role of laboratory information systems on business outcomes in both private and hospital pathology in Australia.

Pathology laboratory information systems are inherently large-scale systems handling large number of data daily to service not only the pathology laboratory itself, but the referring medical practitioners. Patient results are often required in a 'mission critical' timeframe. This research is unique and has not been previously reported.

The following then serves to confirm, through a survey and three focus groups, that pathology laboratories are unable to undertake strategic information system planning (SISP). An organisation achieves the highest stage of strategic information system planning if it possesses an IT/IS strategic plan, fully aligned with business goals, which accurately references, at any point in time, current or target IT themes which provide data of high quality, accuracy, availability, and sharability for informed decisions that will give the organization a competitive advantage. Moreover, this book outlines that the factors that are critical to strategic planning in pathology laboratories in Australia are (a) laboratory information systems capability (b) business–IT alignment (c) strategic spending (d) research and education (e) end-user involvement and (f) information systems effectiveness.

Some of the key findings include that the laboratory information systems are regarded by multiple departments of the health industry as a commodity and therefore are regarded as having no strategic value. This long held view has created a situation whereby pathology as a whole is regarded with little or no priority for funding in hospitals in Australia. In addition, spending in private laboratories is functional and not strategic. Financial considerations provide for internal functional enhancement of the private pathology business that rarely involves the laboratory information systems. Any enhancements to the laboratory information systems are restricted to being functional.

There is a clear distinction between the functionality and the capability of the laboratory information systems. The laboratory information systems lack the capability for integration with, and the use of, modern technology. There is no possibility for the laboratory information systems to complement and enhance the strategic components of such activities as international expansion of private pathology in Australia. There is a lack of pressure within the private pathology industry in particular to take steps to develop the capability of the laboratory information systems which may be attributed to a three-way monopoly in private pathology in Australia. A lack of active research and lack of formal education into management and SISP in the medical and pathology industries is also a contributing factor to the acceptance of the existing status of laboratory information systems capability.

The lack of capability of the laboratory information systems prevents them from fulfilling any strategic role. The ramifications of this are that contributors to successful SISP, such as business–IT alignment, are unable to occur. This then prevents proper SISP, and hence the assessment of information systems effectiveness, to the detriment of business outcomes for pathology in Australia.

It was our goal that this book will provide to the reader a clear picture of a number of issues contributing to a lack of ability of pathology laboratories in Australia to undertake SISP. The research has also highlighted, through the concepts of a hypothesised relationship between SISP and information systems effectiveness measurement, a means and a mechanism for change. The adoption of the principles of this research would assist in the achievement of a more uniform approach to laboratory information systems in Australia that would be beneficial to patients and pathology businesses alike. Changes in pathology laboratory information systems based on the findings of this unique research provide a possible means of contributing to lowering healthcare costs to the nation by increasing internal efficiencies and cost effectiveness of both private and hospital pathology laboratories.

We hope our readers enjoy the journey discovering critical issues central to ICT in a pathology context.

Melbourne, Australia, 2011   Mark Belkin
                                                                                     Brian Corbitt
                                                                        Nilmini Wickramasinghe

References

Wickramasinghe, N., Bali, R., & Schaffer, J. (2008). The health care intelligence continuum: key model for enabling KM initiatives and realizing the full potential of SMT in healthcare delivery. *International Journal of Biomedical Engineering and Technology (IJBET)*, *1*(no. 4), 415–427.

Wickramasinghe, N., Bali, R., Gibbons, C., & Schaffer, J. (2008). Realizing the knowledge spiral in healthcare: the role of data mining and knowledge management. *Studies in Health Technology and Informatics*, *137*, 147–162.

Wickramasinghe, N. (2008). Building a learning healthcare organisation by fostering organisational learning through a process centric view of knowledge management. *International Journal of Innovation and Learning*, *5*(no. 2), 201–216.

Von Lubitz, D., & Wickramasinghe, N. (2006). Networkcentric Healthcare: applying the tools, techniques and strategies of knowledge management to create superior healthcare operations. *International Journal of Electronic Healthcare (IJEH)*, *4*, 415–428

Wickramasinghe, N., Geisler, E., & Schaffer J. (2006). Realizing The value proposition for healthcare by incorporating km strategies and data mining techniques with the use of information communication technologies. *International Journal of Healthcare Technology and Management*, *7*(no. 3/4), 303–318

Wickramasinghe, N., Bali, R. Lehany, B., Gibbons M., & Schaffer, J. (2009). *Healthcare knowledge management primer*. New York: Routledge.

Acknowledgements

This book would not have been possible without the cooperation and assistance of numerous people: many people who provided vital assistance and participated in the research, our institution for affording us the necessary time, our colleagues, students, and the staff at Springer. In addition, we are most appreciative of the support and encouragement provided for our families. Finally, we would especially like to thank the production staff at Springer, in particular Khristine Queja and Kathryn Hiler, for all their efforts in helping us to make this book possible.

Contents

Contributors

Dr Mark Belkin PhD, BAppSc(LabMed) pursued an interest in science and medicine and enrolled in BAppSc (laboratory medicine) at RMIT. He majored in haematology and has worked in the pathology laboratory for 25 + years. Most of his working life was in a senior capacity, and involved clinical, technical, and teaching duties. Dr Belkin enrolled in studies for his PhD (Management Information Systems) at RMIT, and has taught in enterprise systems and BPR, systems integration, and information systems management while studying. His doctoral research was based on a suite of pathology laboratory management programs he designed, and forms the basis of this book. The suite of programs is envisaged to act as a re-engineering tool to change current pathology management structure from a pyramidal hierarchy to a series of laterally linked self contained business units. Dr Belkin currently manages an online medical informatics post graduate course at RMIT and has published in the area of business analysis and strategic planning applied to pathology informatics. He is a member of the Health Informatics Society of Australia.

Professor Brian Corbitt is currently Professor of Information Systems and Deputy Pro Vice Chancellor Business Research at RMIT University. He has previously been Adjunct Professor of IT at KMIT (NB) and then Professor of Management Science at Shinawatra University in Thailand, Pro Vice Chancellor (Online Services at Deakin University, JADE Professor of eCommerce at Victoria University of Wellington in New Zealand) and prior to that lectured at the University of Melbourne, where he was also Head of International House. He specializes in IT policy development, analysis, and implementation, in e-Business Modeling and Electronic Commerce trade relationships, and health policy and IT. He has published 10 books on eBusiness, eCommerce, and eGovernment. He has also published over 150 refereed scholarly papers, and also numerous government reports to the Governments of Thailand and New Zealand, and many invited papers as a keynote speaker on IT policy in Malaysia, Singapore, Thailand, New Zealand, Japan, Hong Kong, and Australia. He is a Senior Editor of Information and Management.

Nilmini Wickramasinghe PhD MBA who currently holds the Epworth Chair Health Information Management, was appointed in Dec 2009 as a Professor to RMIT University's School of Business IT and Logistics after being a professor in the US for 15 years. She researches and teaches in several areas within information systems including knowledge management, e-commerce and m-commerce, and organizational impacts of technology with particular focus on the applications of these areas to healthcare and thereby effecting superior healthcare delivery. Professor Wickramasinghe is well published with more than 200 referred scholarly articles, several books, and an encyclopedia. She has collaborated with many large organizations such as NASA and GE as well as leading healthcare organizations such as the Cleveland Clinic, Johns Hopkins, Kaiser, and NorthWestern Memorial Hospital. In addition, she regularly presents her work throughout North America, as well as in Europe and Australia. Professor Wickramasinghe is the editor-in-chief of two scholarly journals: International Journal of Networking and Virtual Organisations (IJNVO—www.inderscience.com/ijnvo) and International Journal of Biomedical Engineering and Technology (IJBET— www.inderscience.com/ijbet) and the Springer Series editor for Healthcare Delivery in the Information Age.

Chapter 1
Introduction

1.1 Background

This book is concerned with the assessment of medical pathology laboratory information systems effectiveness, and in what way information system effectiveness impacts on the medical pathology business. To achieve this goal we discuss a study that focused on determining the level of Strategic Information Systems Planning (SISP) and by what means information system effectiveness is measured, in private and public hospital pathology laboratories in Australia.

Over the past 20 years medical professionals have increasingly become dependent on the expanding range of sophisticated diagnostic services provided by clinical laboratories (van Merode et al. 1996; Boran et al. 1996; O'Moore et al. 1994; Bossuyt et al. 2007; Friedberg 2008). Automated analytical instruments generate an ever-increasing variety and volume of test information at ever-increasing speeds. In terms of healthcare, this development has been a significant benefit—helping physicians to diagnose and treat illnesses accurately and quickly and to monitor recovery closely (Bender and McNair 1996; Bossuyt et al. 2007).

The modern pathology laboratory, whether private practice or hospital based, is a complex, heterogeneous environment, typically with a mix of autonomous and partially interworking applications running on a range of hardware platforms. A consequence is that bigger laboratories today are entirely dependent on their IT functionality and that the pathology laboratory IT solutions must be considered as 24 h mission critical systems (Bender and McNair 1996; Wells et al. 1996). Most of the current laboratory information systems are mainframe systems, using older software languages and with little flexibility in terms of rapid programming, graphics display, integration with developing technologies and real-time analysis of management data (Boran et al. 1996; Brender and McNair 1996; Belkin et al. 2008 (Appendix A)). The current systems were introduced at the end of the 1960s/early 1970s with the advent of the first auto analysers, which enabled a larger number of tests to be performed in a shorter time period. At this time, the main task that was required of the laboratory information systems was that of a database to store demographics and simple data. Over the next 20 years, the laboratories and the number of tests available expanded

M. Belkin et al., *Strategic ICT Planning in Pathology*,
Healthcare Delivery in the Information Age,
DOI 10.1007/978-1-4614-4478-7_1, © Springer Science+Business Media, LLC 2013

quickly and associated development of laboratory information systems in pathology did not eventuate (Bender and McNair 1996).

Rapid evolution of pathology laboratory procedures, methodologies and equipment characterises the clinical laboratory. The development of pathology laboratory science is so rapid that a vendor organisation has difficulty in absorbing, digesting and practically incorporating new enabling technologies/techniques into their version of a global laboratory information system (Bender and McNair 1996; Boran et al. 1996). Major investment has been made in IT in pathology laboratories, which cannot be ignored. Hence, it is necessary that an IT solution is future viable and able to incorporate already installed IT functionalities (Wells et al. 1996). Experience has shown that within the operation of a laboratory, the processes tend to bend, break or refine the work processes in order to cope with the individual ad hoc service needs (Brender and McNair 1996). The current laboratory business model suffers from fragmentation, redundancy and excess capacity. Such a model has competitive disadvantages and is no longer adequate in the new reality of cost containment and competition (Bossuyt et al. 2007). Information Technology plays a role in overcoming fragmentation, excess capacity and redundancy through consolidation and integration, and contributes to improved cost efficiencies through enhanced diffusion of state-of-the-art-technologies and improved turn-around times (Bossuyt et al. 2007; Porter 2004; Zinn et al. 2001).

The advent of "middleware " as a means to link otherwise incompatible functionalities has grown as an industry in pathology laboratories in Australia and internationally as a result of more stasis in laboratory information systems development in Australia. Middleware is a term used to describe the many different software packages that are available for a variety of information purposes, from a range of vendors including instrument manufacturers (Friedman 2005; Torke et al. 2005). This type of software generally sits between an analyser and the laboratory information system in an ad hoc manner and is required to provide functionality not possible from the laboratory information system alone by linking the analyser to the laboratory information system. The main direction in development of middleware has been auto-verification of patient results and process engineering in an attempt to reduce result turnaround time. Middleware is rapidly expanding in use and functionality and some see it as a replacement for the limited functionality of laboratory information system in its current form (Friedman 2005; Torke et al. 2005).

It is interesting to note in the literature on middleware and its implications that there is no reference made to the design process of middleware and there are apparently no business-oriented components available. There is certainly no consultation between the vendors of the middleware and the potential laboratory users as to the design of the middleware and its supporting information system architecture—this is an example of misalignment in pathology laboratories. Perhaps the benefits of middleware are superficial in the business context and are accepted by the pathology profession because of the perception of a lack of understanding of SISP in pathology laboratories. This perception will also be investigated in this study.

The establishment of open architecture systems implies that a market will develop for modular, scaleable, and cost-effective laboratory information system functionalities, able to be incorporated in a 'plug-and-play' fashion without the dependence on individual manufacturers and hardware/software platforms which characterise current systems. Bender and McNair (1996) and Boran et al. (1996) stressed as one of the main design requirements that the system must be highly flexible and maximally customisable—by the users themselves. More recently, this view has been expanded to indicate that pathology laboratory professionals can differentiate themselves not only by their technical skills but also by being involved in the creation, distribution, and application of knowledge related to laboratory aspects of patient care. Such extra service should be recognised and implemented in the business strategy (Bossuyt et al. 2007; Friedberg 2008).

There has emerged a growing recognition of the relationship between information system facilities and strategic development in pathology laboratories. This was developed in the literature review in terms of the components of SISP, that is, business-IT alignment, cost benefit analysis (financial considerations) and end-user involvement in the planning process. The literature was examined to elucidate those factors influencing the effectiveness of information system in general, and for pathology laboratories in particular, to ascertain the issues relevant to the perceived sub-optimal performance of laboratory information systems and ineffective SISP in pathology laboratories in Australia.

1.2   Problem Domain

The current overall situation of pathology laboratory information systems and management initiated this study. The pathology laboratory community could benefit from a deeper understanding of what is involved in laboratory management, and more specifically, what enables successful SISP and information system effectiveness measurement. An improved understanding of SISP and information system effectiveness measurement may lead laboratory management to more efficiency, improved cost-effectiveness and improved competitive advantage, that is, more positive business outcomes. The focus of this study is both objective (quantitative) and subjective (qualitative). This study was interested to know how the pathology laboratory currently approached its management and information systems development, and what the contras to positive outcomes are. In particular, this study was interested to see if some of, or all of the recognised contras to SISP and information system effectiveness (end-user involvement, business-IT alignment, cost-benefit analysis, UIS) in other business verticals applied to the pathology laboratory. The investigator was interested to know what the pathology laboratory understands of SISP and information system effectiveness measurement—a lack of knowledge of these two processes may be identified as a contra to them in its own right.

In addition to these recognised contras to SISP, the study explored the role of the laboratory information system from the perspective of its functionality along the lines of "task-technology asynchrony", that is, the inability of the laboratory information system to accommodate new and/or enhanced functionality through a lack of technical capability. The role of research and education and its impact on SISP awareness was investigated as a possible significant, but largely overlooked, contra to successful SISP and information system effectiveness. Research and education was investigated in the context that a lack of awareness and knowledge of systems technology and business principles by stakeholders precludes them from being able to contribute to SISP.

1.3 Key Issues

The motivation behind this study is that very little, if any, investigation has been undertaken into information system effectiveness and SISP in pathology. This is thought to have a potentially negative impact on the pathology laboratory as a business. The identification of a source of inadequacy in the planning and assessment processes in SISP and information system effectiveness measurement could be advantageous to the profession, and would enable research and development into processes and procedures to ensure enhanced business outcomes.

There have been studies conducted in an attempt to improve the efficiency and cost effectiveness of pathology laboratories, but these studies do not embrace SISP and some take such approaches as accounting and workflow statistics. Goldschmidt et al. (1998) looked at the functional processes of workstations in the pathology laboratory with the view that staff should be assigned to a workstation when it was active. They proposed coordination of the workflow with the assessment of the state of activity of the workstation and developed planning rules to assign staff to achieve 100 % efficiency. The rules are very complex and require an understanding of advanced mathematics—something well outside the scope of laboratory staff. Their study did not account for redundancy of time, that is, when the laboratory was not busy, and they did not consider the effect or control of peripheral services to the laboratory department, such as specimen delivery.

Revere and Roberts (2004) took more of an accountant's perspective in an attempt at improving cost efficiencies by combining the same services (pathology specimen delivery) of a group of hospitals. Through the use of a modelling process using commercial software, the hospitals were able to develop a seven-day rotating roster—this enabled shorter specimen delivery times to the hospital laboratory that in turn shortened turnaround times for results. The exercise also saved 16.4 % per annum in courier wages.

Mayer (1998) also took a financial approach to improving cost efficiencies in pathology laboratories with the use of commercially available cost analysis software. The software is a management tool that compares costs of procedures and activities. This information could then be used for evaluation of operations and decision making for the laboratory.

These studies, which consider only one aspect of the overall management of a laboratory (business), are time consuming and require outside skills to perform. They do not align with any SISP components and do not consider other aspects of the planning process. They may therefore be regarded as functional and not strategic studies. It is significant that with these three approaches, outside software and specialised people were required to develop and perform the processes, and that laboratory staff in general were not consulted or involved in the planning process. The OpenLabs project (Boran et al. 1996), on the other hand, approached the problem of an information system change from the SISP process perspective. The consortium members included partners from industry, academia and laboratory services and they worked as a close-knit team to develop specifically identified and detailed change items. In the process used by the OpenLabs consortium, such SISP components as end-user involvement, business-IT alignment and pre-planning partnering were applied to ensure a successful outcome. The measure of success of the OpenLabs project was measured by the achievement of the original business objectives (Boran et al. 1996; O'Moore et al. 1994).

The investigator explored and reported on the reasons why there is not a broader approach to SISP and information system effectiveness measurement in pathology laboratories, paying particular attention to the role of the existing laboratory information system. This book will therefore explore key questions including:

How does the effectiveness of laboratory information systems impact on business outcomes in medical pathology practice?
Does SISP occur in pathology in Australia?
What are the determinants of information system effectiveness in pathology laboratories in Australia?

The investigation has identified the components of effective systems planning in pathology practice and gained a better understanding of the elements involved and their effect on business outcomes for pathology practices. It was of particular interest to the investigator to understand by what means a pathology laboratory information system is deemed effective in pathology laboratory practice, this interest having arisen from his criticism of current methods of assessing information system effectiveness as seen in the literature (Belkin et al. 2008). This study provides the potential, through the gaining of these insights, to develop a more standardised approach to SISP and information system effectiveness measurement in pathology laboratories in Australia. Given the important role for IS/IT in enabling and supporting superior healthcare delivery as well as the key function that pathology plays in effecting successful healthcare diagnosis and subsequent treatment, we believe it is vital to focus attention on the role for IS/IT with regard to pathology laboratory practice and we believe our readers will also realise the importance and significance of this research area on reading the following material.

Chapter 2
SISP and IS Effectiveness

2.1 Introduction

Reviewing SISP experience throughout years of practice provides the knowledge base upon which to define the research model and test hypotheses. The internal and external environments of SISP are analysed in this chapter to better understand the constructs relevant for the scope of this study.

Today's information rich and knowledge-based business society relies heavily on Information Technology (IT) (Wang and Tai 2003) and Information Systems (Rondeau et al. 2006; Wickramasinghe et al. 2009). The IT and information systems are designed to enable the business to operate effectively and hopefully create a competitive advantage. Firms gain benefit from aligning their information systems design and performance with the core business competencies and business goals of the firm (Grover and Segars 2005; Burn and Szeto 2000; Chan et. al. 1997; King 1998). There are multiple paths towards this end and inefficiencies and conflicts may arise when the firm's information systems strategies diverge from the business goals (Rondeau et al. 2006). This is no different in the health industry where conflicts exist between information systems infrastructure and development, and business goals—that is to say, there is business-IT misalignment. The existence of inflexible mainframe based file sharing information systems that are unable to support modern technology, such as the Internet, telemedicine, wireless technology and real-time management software, and which suffer poor performance under load has compromised the business goals and business development in the health vertical to the extent that it has now fallen behind other comparable knowledge industries (Wells et al. 1996; Kaplan 1987; Bossuyt et al. 2007).

There are a variety of approaches in the literature that try to overcome the problem of misalignment to improve the efficiency of the design process. Hackney et al. (1999) suggest that misalignment in information systems strategies, goals, and objectives may be avoided by increasing end-user involvement. Gerwin and Kolodny (1992) regard the implementation of cross-functional decision processes as a means to the promotion of interdependent work. This is typically achieved through the creation of greater work system integration. Cross-functional decision practices are infrequently referred to in the literature (Gerwin and Kolodny 1992) and this implies

M. Belkin et al., *Strategic ICT Planning in Pathology*,
Healthcare Delivery in the Information Age,
DOI 10.1007/978-1-4614-4478-7_2, © Springer Science+Business Media, LLC 2013

a degree of single vision on the part of researchers when they refer to the planning process.

Where reference is made to more cohesiveness between information systems capability, independence of the information systems department and the alignment of business goals, there is no mechanism or detail given on how this is achieved. Grover and Segars (2005) claim that while there have been studies that examine the "what" questions in SISP, particularly concerning the issue of business–information systems alignment, there has been little on the "how" questions, which include the process of planning and whether this yields effective outcomes. The presumption that businesses will change their planning processes over time in an attempt to improve their effectiveness and leverage their investment in SISP is also raised.

In this study, SISP is investigated through the concept of a system that is defined by its behaviour, structure and evolution. Special emphasis is placed on the evolution and structure of SISP to find relevant constructs for assessing SISP. Important SISP constructs such as SISP approaches, methods, techniques and tools are critically assessed. Several other SISP constructs like alignment of SISP and business, and key stakeholders are discussed with respect to the key reasons for SISP success/failure.

SISP behaviour, structure and evolution are described to provide the grounding material for defining the hypothesis and to demonstrate the gap in the existing knowledge to be addressed by this research. This will indicate how the research question *"How does the effectiveness of laboratory information systems impact on business outcomes in medical pathology practice?"* was developed.

2.2 Strategic Information Systems Planning (SISP)

Strategic Information System Planning (SISP) has evolved in method and style over the last decade on the basis that it emphasises the need to bring IT to align with and sometimes influence the strategic direction of the firm. In rich IT environments this has a recognised relevance to competitiveness (Grover and Segars 2005). The degree to which IT aligns with the strategic direction of medical pathology private and hospital practice and the resulting impact on competitiveness of medical pathology practices will be evaluated in this research. An approach to the investigation of this relationship will be determined in Chap. 3.

With the more recent proliferation of Internet-based computing, outsourcing, personal computers and user applications, the trend is to push developmental activities outside the exclusive domain of professional information systems groups thus creating challengers that did not exist when SISP was first conceived. This has evolved into a proactive search by many firms for competitive and value-adding opportunities co-existing with the development of broad policies and procedures for integrating, co-ordinating, controlling and implementing the IT resource (Grover and Segars 2005).

However, although much has been studied with respect to business and IT alignment, little research has been undertaken into the mechanisms of SISP, including process planning. Grover and Segars (2005) examined the evolution and maturing of SISP from the early 1970s and made several important observations. The work conducted in the 1970s was later supported by other researchers such as Sullivan (1985), Earl (1993), and Sabherwal and King (1995). Grover and Segars (2005) found that many studies focused on planning content with particular interest in methods and measurement of alignment between business and IS strategy (Burn and Szeto 2000; Chan et al. 1997; King 1988). Grover and Segars (2005) observed that these studies did little to illuminate the organisational aspects of planning. Early studies by Pyburn (1983), in an attempt to identify institutionalised planning dimensions, actions and behaviours, made field observations which noted the existence of both a rational/structured process and a personal/informal process.

Earl (1993) made similar observations when he distinguished SISP approaches based on the degree of rationality and adaptability built into the planning process. Earl (1993) however, noted a hybrid organisational system of planning which seemed to be more effective than the highly structured and less adaptable rational approaches. This observation was ratified by the work of Sullivan (1985) and Sabherwal and King (1995). Further research by several authors (Boynton and Zmud 1987; Zmud et al. 1986 and Lederer and Sethi 1998) has also implied that such systems may be necessary in order to manage increasingly diverse and dispersed technologies across the organisation.

2.2.1   SISP Stages of Growth Models

Evolution, or stages of growth models, is popular in organisational research and information systems planning. The best known of these being perhaps Nolan's stages of growth model (Nolan 1979). In this model (Fig. 2.1) Nolan proposed that the growth of computing follows an S-shaped curve through a preliminary phase in which planning procedures are beginning to be defined, an evolving stage in which planning activities are tested but still being defined and a mature stage in which procedures are in place. In terms of the experience of the operatives, the preliminary stage implies little or no planning experience, the evolving stage implies some experience and the mature stage implies a history of planning activities and much experience in the hands of participants. The suggestion that shifting the emphasis from "descriptive" to "prescriptive" can more effectively plan for and organise the computing recourse based on predictable stages is made by Nolan.

Nolan's (1979) hypothesis has been controversial and is perhaps dated for today's technological context (Grover and Segars 2005). There is, however, a key implication that should be noted. Nolan (1979) suggested that his model could be viewed as a learning model where movement through the stages is influenced by the environment (changing technology) and the adaptation to that environment by internal adjustments—ultimately the stage of 'maturity' systems naturally mirror their context. Nolan's model has a degree of bi-directionality about it and has an in-built means for change management, placing it apart from the myriad of

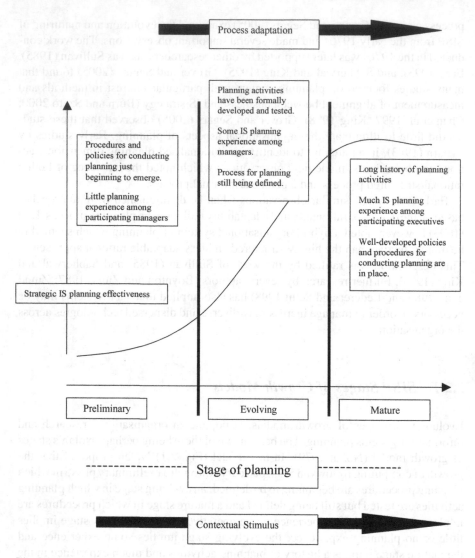

Fig. 2.1 Strategic information systems planning model. (Adapted from Nolan 1979)

uni-directional models derived by other authors (Wang and Tai 2003; Grover et al. 1996).

Porter and Millar (1985) used the life cycle concept to illustrate how industries develop and how businesses adapt to pressure. Greiner (1972) described a model in which firms grew based on learning from crisis. Applegate et al. (1996) describe technology assimilation in firms that evolved through stages of "slack and control" to learn how to use new technologies more effectively. Magal et al. (1998) indicated that information centres evolved by adapting and learning from their client base, ultimately being treated as a major corporate resource. Henderson et al. (1987) also described their stages of end-user computing as a learning curve.

There is a common thread in the approaches of all of these authors in that their planning is based on undertaking a planning exercise with little prior experience, learning from crisis and mistakes, being influenced by external client factors and a 'change as we go' attitude. One would think that this approach is counterproductive due to time lost in learning and sorting mistakes—any competitive advantage through information systems planning and technology could be lost. The planning process may be made more effective by way of more intense business analysis to define and align the information systems parameters. A means of evaluating the resultant information systems is also required (Irani and Love 2001).

2.2.2   Information Systems Evaluation

The difficulties in measuring benefits and costs of information systems are often the cause of uncertainty about the expected impact of information systems and thus, are major problems faced by the decision-makers. As a result, the information systems evaluation process is often ignored, or ineffectively or inefficiently carried out. The reason for this is that managers consider the evaluation process takes too long, costs a significant amount of money with little visible return, and involves too many people with departmental or individual political agendas (Irani and Love 2001). Approaching any evaluative activity, we need to consider the context of evaluation (who is evaluating and why), the process (how) and the content (what; Symons 1991). This is even more so in the field of health informatics where the traditions of medicine meet and interact with the information systems field (Klecun and Cornford 2005).

As an example of evaluation difficulties in health informatics, we can consider the UK health sector. Policy has proposed over a number of years and formulations that information and communications technology can serve as a fundamental driver for reform and modernisation of the National Health Service (NHS) (DOH 1997, 2002). The situation becomes yet more challenging when an organisation, such as the NHS, is engaged in a range of complementary or interdependent change programs at the same time, and the consequences and outcomes of any particular project cannot be isolated from all the other changes taking place (Klecun and Cornford 2005). Many contemporary health information systems are complex and aim to be both technologically and organisationally innovative, involving a large number of different stakeholders, spanning institutions and professions, and (potentially) changing both the way people and organisations work and the ways in which services are delivered and experienced (Klecun and Cornford 2005).

Against this background, it is not surprising that evaluation, although discussed extensively in both the information systems and health informatics literature, remains controversial and in practice often stumbles into trouble (Klecun and Cornford 2005). Many accounts indicate how it can be incomplete, biased or just 'touching the

surface' (Smithson and Hirschheim 1998; Farbey et. al. 1999). Traditionally, evaluation of information systems has become focused on technical aspects of a system, its
performance, reliability, robustness and security, cost-benefit, and immediate questions of usability. As information systems have become more pervasive, ambitious,
complex and interactive, evaluation emphasis has, to a degree, shifted to concerns
with how and to what extent information system innovations serve ambitions of
organisational change (Klecun and Cornford 2005). This in turn leads to political,
cultural and organisational aspects being seen as necessarily playing a major role
in shaping the evaluation activity (Walsham 1993). Thus, issues of alignment with
business goals and institutional interests, understanding of existing work practices in
formal and informal senses, and the diverse power bases and competing stakeholder
groups and their information needs, have all been given attention in the information
systems field (Symons 1991; Smithson and Hirschheim 1998).

The implementation and maintenance of information systems is invariably a costly
exercise for organisations, so it is only natural for managers to assume that they should
provide their organisation with a degree of economic value (Irani and Love 2001).
McKay and Marshall (2001) express concern that managers do not perceive that they
are deriving value for money when it comes to information systems investments.
Organisations continue to report that the deployment of information systems within
their organisation has resulted in the substitution of old problems with new ones
(techno-based; Irani and Love 2001). In addition, the introduction of information
systems can be a huge disappointment, since unexpected difficulties and failures are
regularly encountered with expected business benefits often not realised (McKay and
Marshall 2001). Furthermore, the human cost of information systems failure (such
as not realising stakeholder expectations) can be quite considerable, and prevent the
take-up of future technology, thus impacting the long-term survival and growth of
the business (Irani and Love 2001).

According to McKay and Marshall (2001), there appears to be a dichotomy with
respect to the question of investment in information systems. On the one hand, the
notion of an information-based economy and the arrival of an e-business domain have
led to considerable faith being placed in information technology to deliver performance improvements. On the other hand, there is concern that information systems
are not delivering what was promised by vendors and project champions. Irani and
Love (2001) attribute this lack of delivery to the difficulty in determining business
value from information systems investments, and the considerable indirect costs associated with enterprise-wide systems. Klecun and Cornford (2005) raise the issue
of information systems success meaning different things to different stakeholders,
further complicating attempts at objective evaluation.

To add to the complication of information systems evaluation, there remains a
host of tools and techniques available to managers for the purpose of information
systems appraisal (*ex-ante* evaluation). Yet, there has been a lack of consensus in
defining and measuring information systems investments (Renkema and Berghout
1997; Irani and Love 2002). Research studies report contradictory findings on the
relationship between information systems investments and organisation productivity
and performance (Grover et al 1998; Bannister and Remenyi 2000). Considering

the growing needs for business to gain a competitive advantage in their respective marketplaces, the evaluation of technical innovations (E-Government, Enterprise Application Integration, E-commerce and Customer Relationship Management) will remain a necessity if the benefits of information systems are to be fully realised. Viewed in systems terms, evaluation provides the basic feedback function to managers as well as forming a fundamental component of the organisational learning process (Smithson and Hirschheim 1998). Evaluation provides the benchmarks of what is to be achieved by the IT/information systems investment. While these benchmarks can later be used to provide a measure of the actual implementation success of information systems projects (Irani and Love 2001), it is worthwhile at this stage of this literature review to consider the prior events to implementation, that is, the planning process. A cohesive and structured planning process lays the platform for development of information systems and, as will be argued in this literature review, successful project development is unlikely to succeed without it.

2.2.3   Planning Process Dimensions and Contexts of SISP

More recent studies by Grover and Segars (1998, 2005) described and measured planning process dimensions and found hybrid systems tended to be more successful and seemed to apply generally to a variety of industries. Through their research, Grover and Segars (2005) identified six important process dimensions of SISP: comprehensiveness; formalisation; focus; flow; participation; and consistency. These dimensions are robust in describing the SISP design and extend beyond the methodological-based and less generalisable descriptions of planning. The authors comment that as organisations become technologically and geographically complex, the importance of planning activities increases. As a result, they argue that a planning culture may emerge in the form of highly structured systems. Rationality may be built into strategic planning systems through higher levels of formalisation, a focus on control and top-down planning flow.

Adaptability refers to the capability of the planning system to learn. The planning system should contain characteristics that will alert managers to changing organisational and environmental conditions that may require a change in strategy. Adaptability may be designed into a system through wide participation profiles (Baets 1992) and through higher levels of planning consistency (Eisenhardt 1989). Such characteristics reflect the importance of gathering information from a number of sources and the importance of consistently reconciling strategic decisions with environmental conditions.

Wang and Tai (2003) add to the process dimensions for success in SISP with their work on organisational contexts, commenting that most process-oriented research has recommended using integration and implementation mechanisms while not considering the possible contingent effect of contextual factors. They suggest that this may lead to the planning system being less adaptable to different organisational contexts and therefore be overly deterministic. Wang and Tai's (2003) model is an

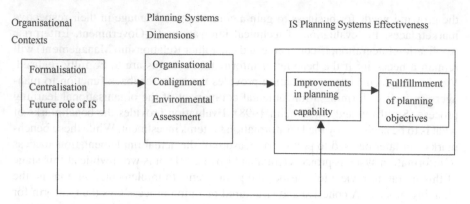

Organisational   Planning Systems   IS Planning Systems Effectiveness
Contexts   Dimensions

Fig. 2.2 Conceptual model—contextual factors role in SISP effectiveness. (Adapted from Wang and Tai 2003)

attempt to integrate organisational contexts into SISP. This can be seen in Fig. 2.2 below.

This conceptual model of Wang and Tai (2003) has three domains:

• Organisational contexts—this domain deals with organisational factors such as formalisation, centralisation and the future role of information systems.
• Planning system dimensions—this domain consists of two categories: organisational co-alignment and environmental assessment. Organisational co-alignment reflects the internal alignment among the four organisational factors (resources committed to planning, implementation mechanisms, acceptance of planning and integration mechanisms) having a strong influence on an organisation's information systems planning and effectiveness, whereas environmental assessment captures the orientation of the planning system.
• Information systems planning system effectiveness—this domain has two parts— the improvements in planning capability and the extent to which the planning system objectives are fulfilled.

Overall, the study by Wang and Tai (2003) holds that organisational contexts can impact the effectiveness of information systems planning indirectly through mediating effects of the planning system's dimensions while these dimensions can influence the improvements in planning capability directly and the fulfillment of planning objectives indirectly. "Resources committed to planning" and "acceptance of planning" (Wang and Tai 2003) together should reflect the organisational support to information systems planning activities, and are similar to the "favourable organisational context of planning" suggested by Steiner (1979). "Integration mechanisms" are the methods used to integrate business goals and plans into information systems strategies and possible mechanisms include the participation of information systems managers in strategic business planning and active interaction between information systems and business planners. "Implementation mechanisms" are the efforts to overcome problems, such as management control systems for review and feedback, resource mobilisation for implementing the plans and top management and user involvement in monitoring implementation (Doll 1985). Consistent with a prior study (Venkatraman and Ramanujaman 1987), the improvements in planning capability can affect the fulfillment of planning objectives.

Wang and Tai (2003) acknowledge that although their work is generally supported by empirical data, a theory of information systems planning is currently lacking. Their results did however support the contention that information systems planning is a rational-adaptive process, supporting the arguments of Pyburn (1983), Earl (1993), Sabherwal and King (1995), and Grover and Segars (2005). Having discussed the process dimension and contexts of SISP, it is now appropriate to consider by what means information systems effectiveness is measured.

2.2.4   Information Systems Effectiveness Indicators

The link between strategic performance and planning has been found to be inconsistent by several authors (Grover and Segars 2005; Raghunathan and Raghunathan 1988). Premkumar and King (1992) on the other hand found that firms in which information systems play a critical role have higher levels of planning resources and are more effective at planning. Medical pathology practices, both private and hospital based, require a mission critical status from their laboratory information systems for the provision of patients services. The literature pertaining to the level of planning resource deployment and planning effectiveness will be examined in Chap. 3, as a basis for further investigation by this research. Lederer and Sethi (1988) explain this relationship by identifying a variety of inhibitors from failure to consider business strategy to time span and resources. The measurement of effectiveness of information systems has been too uni-dimensional (such as financial ratios; Rubin 2004), measured on a single item scale or focused on limited aspects of planning, such as alignment with business strategy only to be comprehensive in assessment of information systems effectiveness.

Other indicators suggested for assessment of information systems effectiveness have been information systems usage, user information satisfaction (UIS), quality of decision making, productivity from cost/benefit analysis and system quality (Ein-Dor and Segev 1978). UIS is described by Petter et al. (2008) as the users' level of satisfaction with reports, websites and support services. The most commonly favoured factors have been information systems use and UIS; because of a lack of a theoretical framework for placing UIS within the greater context of overall 'information systems effectiveness ', its relevance as a performance measurement has been questioned (Grover et al. 1996). Gation (1994, p. 119) elaborates on the context position of UIS as a surrogate measure of information systems effectiveness by saying "If an effective system is defined as one that adds value to the firm, then an effective system must have some positive influence on user behaviour (i.e. must improve productivity, decision making and so on). Advocates of UIS argue that there is some theoretical support for linking attitudes (i.e. satisfaction) and behaviour in the "psychology literature".

The questionable relevance of UIS as a performance measurement has been demonstrated in one instance in the laboratory experiment conducted by Yuthas and Young (1998) on materials management information systems in which they investigated the relationship between management performance, user satisfaction and system usage. The study involved the development of a computerised inventory system which was used by 59 undergraduate business students assuming the role of a materials manager for a small catering company dealing with highly perishable inventory. The task required of subjects was to prepare a purchase order for the company's anticipated inventory needs for one day. In order to assist the subjects in performing the task, written and system reports were provided. Four measures of effectiveness were used: decision-making performance; user satisfaction; system usage time and system usage volume report. In the course of executing their tasks, the would-be managers observed that information systems plays a vital role in the materials management function by providing timely and accurate information necessary for the accomplishment of decision-making goals (Yuthas and Young 1998).

This information includes inventory control, purchasing, electronic data interchange, master production scheduling, capacity management, production activity control and materials requirements planning. Materials managers use systems to monitor their stock status, to alert themselves to critical shortages and to trigger purchase orders when reorder points are reached. The managers rely heavily on these reports, often consulting these information sources rather than touring the warehouse. Managers must be able to ascertain whether and to what extent information systems are assisting to achieve decision-making goals, such as reduction of inventory costs.

Yuthas and Young (1998) found that correlations among the three measures suggest that although satisfaction and usage are closely associated with performance, the relationships among the measures were not sufficiently strong to warrant their usage as interchangeable measures of effectiveness. That is, high levels of satisfaction and system use do not guarantee that the system actually increases management effectiveness. These authors hold the view that because information systems are generally designed to provide information to support decision making, decision performance is the most direct measure of effectiveness. Yuthas and Young (1998) suggest direct measures, such as turnover, fill-rates and inventory costs, as being appropriate measures of information systems effectiveness in materials management; this would suggest that the information system is better aligned with the business goals of the firm to maintain competitive advantage. Importantly, Yuthas and Young (1998) also comment on the role of management support and proper training of all users as an adjunct to effective use of information systems. This suggests a rather functional, hands-on view of the measurement of information systems effectiveness.

Grover and Segars (2005), by contrast, have a more strategic view with their development of a multidimensional conceptualisation of five key dimensions of SISP effectiveness, which recognise that there are outcomes that can be directly expected from a good planning system. The authors also recognise that SISP is a complex activity with a variety of benefits, and the contribution of SISP captured in terms of bottom line figures, such as return on investment (ROI) and return on equity (ROE), may be significantly confounded by many uncontrolled business, economic and environmental factors. Grover and Segars (2005) also argue that successful SISP should achieve alignment between information systems and business strategy; analyse and understand the business and associated technologies; foster cooperation and partnership between managers and user groups; anticipate relevant events/issues within the competitive environment and adapt to unexpected organisational and environmental change. Grover and Segars (2005) also argue a fundamental proposition that SISP will adapt over time through redesign of its process dimensions and that this redesign will result in more effective SISP. This multidimensional conceptualisation approach supports previous arguments by Weill and Olsen (1989) and Delone and McLean (1992). The author's approach also infers the capacity for the multidimensional model to be fluid and dynamic and ongoing. However, all the cited authors acknowledge that further research is needed to define the construct space for effectiveness criteria, as discussed below.

2.2.5 *Construct Model for IS Effectiveness*

Delone and McLean (1992, 2003) have focused on effectiveness with their information systems success model. The model consists of six interdependent constructs: system quality; information quality; use; user satisfaction; individual impact; and organisational impact. The basis for this model is product oriented. For example, system quality describes measures of the information processing system. Information quality represents measures of information systems output—typically the measures in this area include accuracy, precision, currency, timeliness and reliability of information provided. An earlier study (Mason 1978) labeled these two categories as production and product respectively. The model implies the measurement of overall success based on items arbitrarily selected from one construct is likely to be inaccurate. Instead, the measure of overall success should combine individual measures from these constructs to create a comprehensive scheme for performance.

Grover et al. (1996) have developed a theoretically based construct space for information systems effectiveness, which complements the information systems success model of Delone and McLean (1992). Grover et al.'s (1996) construct model provides a means of cross-validating the information systems success model and they attempt to synthesize the seemingly disparate array of effectiveness measures and research approaches through definitional dimensions of evaluative referent, unit of analysis and evaluation type. The evaluative referent describes the relative standard that is used as a basis for assessing performance. Combining these perspectives with the others found in studies (Hamilton and Chervany 1981; Ives et al. 1983), three potential evaluative judgments emerge: comparative, normative and improvement. The evaluative perspective of comparative judgment attempts to compare the effectiveness of a particular system with other 'similar' systems—typically those set up in similar organisations. A typical question in this mode is—How does our system's performance compare with similar systems in comparable organisations? Although this perspective is intuitive, it may be difficult to actually implement. Gathering timely and accurate information regarding comparable systems is very difficult.

Within the perspective of normative judgment, a relevant assessment question is—How does our system's performance compare against that of a theoretically ideal system? In fact, the system is compared to 'systems of best practice' rather than those of an organisation. This approach is amenable to research contexts providing the literature and experts readily identify the 'standards'.

The third perspective of improvement judgment can be summarised by the following relevant question—How much have the capabilities of the system improved over time? The focus is therefore on assessing how information systems has evolved or improved (over time) in supporting organisational needs. Grover et al. (1996) are of the opinion that this third perspective is useful in cases where the system is in its initial stages and has yet to reach steady state. This opinion suggests conflict with the actual relevant question of improvement with time—steady state suggests an equilibrium with constant indices and raises the question of lack of capacity for change—an essential form of information systems effectiveness. To build a complete picture of information systems effectiveness, evaluation must be conducted from both a macro (organisational) and micro (individual) view. Such evaluation is necessary because information systems supports individual as well as organisational decision-making and can also provide competitive advantage (Grover et al. 1996).

From the organisational effectiveness literature, Brewer (1983) argues that there are three types of evaluation: process; response; and impact. Process evaluation involves the assumption that organisational members work to ensure efficient use of resources when resources are limited. This assessment is based on user dependence on information systems, user perceptions of system ownership and the extent to which an information systems is disseminated throughout organisational administration and operating procedure (Trice and Treacy 1986).

Response evaluation assesses the individual or the organisation to the information systems service or product. This assessment has significance in respect to user resistance to innovation and implementation. Any resistance or habitualisation must be identified to ensure successful implementation. This assessment also considers complex variables such as user's beliefs and attitudes toward information systems in general which are important for fulfillment of information system planning (Grover et al. 1996).

Impact evaluation represents the most comprehensive and most difficult to assess evaluation. It is associated with the direct effects of information systems implementation on the individual and/or the organisation. Grover et al. (1996) derived the following model (Fig. 2.3) consisting of six classes of information systems effectiveness measurement, which define the overall construct space for information systems effectiveness.

As shown in the Grover et al. (1996) model, the evaluation of information systems is initiated by choice of the relevant evaluative referent, which describes the relative standard that is used as a basis for assessing performance. The first three classes of effectiveness measures are associated with macro (organisational) evaluation. From their empirical work developing this model, Grover et al. (1996, p. 182) state "in

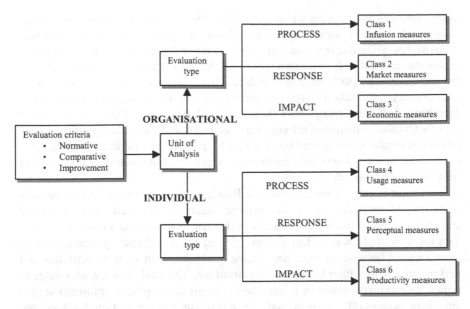

Fig. 2.3 The construct space for information systems effectiveness. (Based on Grover et al. 1996)

general, it seems that both theoretical depictions strongly imply that information systems effectiveness is multidimensional in terms of types of measures and level of analysis." This statement supports their earlier stated contention, and supports the argument of other authors (Earl 1993; Pyburn 1983; Sullivan 1985).

2.2.6   *Information Systems Evaluation Perspective*

The multidimensional approach of Grover and Segars (1996) may be regarded as an evolution of the Delone and McLean (1992) information systems success model, which considered six interdependent constructs (system quality, information quality, use, user satisfaction, individual impact and organisation impact) in a more uni-dimensional context. As stated earlier (Chap. 2, p. 19), the measurement of overall success based on items arbitrarily selected from one construct is likely to be inaccurate.

Brewer (1983) has the view that process evaluation involves the assumption that organisational members work to ensure efficient use of resources, the assumption being based on user dependence on information technology and user perceptions of ownership. Saarinen (1996) raises the issues of correctness of interpretation of information systems, effectiveness measures and personal bias in information systems product evaluation (Chap. 2, p. 30). These personal issues should be addressed in the context of full and proper evaluation of information systems products and developments. Further discourse by Grover et al. (1996) on evaluation perspective rightly raises questions asking from whose perspective the evaluation is being carried out. Though information systems may be viewed as effective from one standpoint, it may be viewed as ineffective from another. Cameron and Whetten (1983) suggest that one reason that no 'best' criterion exists is because there is no 'best' constituency. Hamilton and Chervany (1981) refer to four different viewpoints on information systems effectiveness: information systems personnel, users, management and internal audit. Members of all these groups have their parochial viewpoints. Grover et al. (1996) state that for the evaluation of information systems effectiveness, the specific views of all groups should be considered because they help to increase awareness of the value of the information systems and help the understanding of the multidimensionality of information systems effectiveness.

This view is ratified by the work of Rondeau et al. (2006) who undertook a study into information systems management effectiveness and end-user computing and its impact on information systems performance in manufacturing firms. The data for their study was collected from 256 senior manufacturing managers who were selected because of their perspective on information systems activities and performance within their respective organisations. The study framework relates to organisational involvement in information systems development, information systems management effectiveness, end-user self reliance in application development, end-user dependence on information systems expertise and information systems performance. Information systems management effectiveness is assessed by three elements: information systems strategic planning effectiveness, information systems responsiveness to organisational computing demands, and information systems effectiveness in end-user training.

The Rondeau et al. (2006) study showed that managers can create an environment that fosters cooperation and teamwork toward organisational rather than functional goals but in many firms, the relationship has been framed in an adversarial manner. They also comment that if the information systems unit asserts its authority to make the rules without the participation and cooperation of the other business units, end-users will continue to break them. Rondeau et al. (2006) also found that if organisations can create an atmosphere of mutual respect and cooperation among these units for the common good of the firm, information systems resources will be highly valued and effectively used and end-user perceptions of information systems performance will increase. Their study concluded that the significant improvements resulting from a better relationship between the information systems unit and end-users were increased information systems strategic planning effectiveness, more highly responsive and better designed computing solutions, and more useful end-user training programs.

The findings of the study by Rondeau et al. (2006) ratify Hackney et al.'s (1999) earlier views on the significance of end-user involvement in planning. Hackney et al. (1999) hold the view that the information-based society requires firms to develop information systems that are flexible, integrative, responsive, and information rich. Firms must align their information systems unit with core business procedures; multiple paths toward strategic alignment can exist and conflicts may arise when a firm's information systems technology strategies exceed its ability to align them with its business strategy. Misalignment of information systems strategies, goals and objectives may be avoided by increasing end-user involvement (Hackney and Kawalek 1999). Increased end-user involvement together with better alignment of business and IT may create a greater holistic organisational approach to management, the ramifications of which are described in the following section.

2.2.7   Cross-functional Decision Process and Information Systems Management Practices

Greater organisational involvement in information systems planning processes creates a better fit with the information systems requirements of a firm operating in an information-rich society. The implementation of cross-functional decision processes creates greater work system integration, collapses traditional organisational boundaries, and promotes independent work (Gerwin and Kolodny 1992). With greater organisational involvement comes a revised set of information systems management practices that better fit the information systems requirements of a firm operating in an information-rich society. The result is improved information systems management effectiveness. Bhattacherjee (2001) makes the point that when information systems management is viewed as highly effective, users are more likely to report greater satisfaction with their systems and to exhibit high levels of information systems performance.

The study of Rondeau et al. (2006) explored the relationship between the information systems unit and the end-user in the context of organisational involvement in information systems related activities. Their study provided valid and reliable measures for end-user involvement related activities, cross-functional involvement in information systems related activities, information systems strategic planning effectiveness, information systems responsiveness to organisational computing demands, end-user self-reliance in application development, and end-user dependence on information systems expertise. The authors comment that managers can create an environment of greater organisational involvement that can only result in a better performing information systems unit that users will value and depend on to provide information services to the firm. A number of decision processes and management practices have been examined and the following section assesses methods of implementation of these processes and practices.

2.2.8   Means and Methods of Information Systems Effectiveness Measurement

Grover et al. (1996) found that a number of criteria are still used to assess information systems effectiveness. Of the criteria used, UIS was most used, followed by usage, cost/benefit analysis, firm performance, user attitudes and value perception.

Gatian (1994) provides some insights into UIS in its role as a surrogate measure of information systems effectiveness. If an effective system is defined as one that adds value to the firm, then an effective system must have some positive influence on user behaviour (for instance—improve productivity, decision-making). Advocates of UIS argue that there is theoretical support for linking attitudes (i.e. satisfaction) and behaviour in the psychological literature. Many researchers and practitioners agree that emphasis in information systems research has shifted from efficiency measures towards effectiveness measures, including user perceived effectiveness measures such as user satisfaction (Srinivasan 1985). Increasing use of UIS questionnaires in firms as a measure of system effectiveness is further evidence of this shift (Conrath and Mignen 1990; Davis 1989).

In the information systems literature, two primary reasons for this shift towards UIS in particular are frequently mentioned. Firstly, many believe in the psychological expectancy theory that attitudes (i.e. satisfaction) are linked to behaviour (i.e. productivity; Fishbein 1967; Fishbein and Ajzen 1975). More to the point, it is believed that satisfied users will be more productive. The second reason for moving away from efficiency measures is that it has traditionally been more difficult to measure white-collar efficiency or productivity directly. If an effective system is one that adds value to the firm, any measure of system effectiveness should reflect some positive change in user behaviour, that is, improved productivity, fewer errors or better decision-making. The use of UIS as a measure of information systems effectiveness, however, still attracts discussion by academics. The following section examines some of this discussion in more detail.

2.2.9 Shortcomings of Evaluation Criteria for Information Systems Effectiveness Measurement

The implicit assumption made by managers and researchers employing UIS questionnaires for system effectiveness evaluation is that satisfied users will perform better than users with poor or neutral attitudes (Bailey and Pearson 1983). Gation (1994) points out the controversial nature of this view given that there is little information in the literature linking user satisfaction with any measures of user behaviour. There is one possible exception to this being research attempting to link satisfaction with system usage, system usage not necessarily translating to improved productivity or effectiveness, especially where usage is mandatory (Gation 1994).

Gation (1994) also rightly raises the still pertinent question of proper and relevant question selection, and the possibility of careless interpretation of results leading to the drawing of poor conclusions. In her study to determine the validity of UIS as a measure of information systems effectiveness, Gation (1994) looked at the relationship between user satisfaction and user performance for a particular system. Within the limitations of the study, user satisfaction is correlated with two measures of performance—the system affected decision-making performance of users and the system affected user efficiency. The research focused on users of college and

university information systems at 39 different campuses. Two groups were studied—
staff in the controller's office who were direct users and academic department heads
who were indirect users. Both groups were asked to assess, via questionnaire, their
own satisfaction and impact of the information system on their own decision-making
performance.

The study overall supported the validity of UIS as a measure of information systems effectiveness. Specifically, the following relationships were revealed between
both user groups. Firstly, a relationship between UIS and decision performance supported the psychological theory that availability of relevant information improves
decision performance in a modern information systems setting. Secondly, a relationship between UIS and information systems efficiency provided support for the
construct UIS as a measure of information systems effectiveness, suggesting that
satisfied users may be more productive (Gation 1994).

It is interesting to note that, in the selection of suitable criteria for measurement
of information systems effectiveness, UIS is still regarded as a key criterion in this
role. It would appear that one of the main objections to this is that UIS as a criterion
of information systems effectiveness has little relationship with the primary business
goals of the firm and hence questionable strategic significance (Grover et al. 1996;
Saarinen 1996). Petter, DeLone and McLean (2008) have recently revisited the role of
UIS instruments as a measure of information systems effectiveness in their extensive
review of the literature pertaining to measuring information systems success. They
compared the Doll et al. (1994) End-User Computing Support (EUCS) instrument
and the Ives et al. (1983) User Information Satisfaction (UIS) instrument and found
the EUCS instrument outperformed the UIS instrument in the context of accounting.
They point out that both the EUCS and UIS instruments contain items relating to
system quality, information quality and service quality, rather than only measuring
overall user satisfaction with the system. Because of this, some researchers have
chosen to parse out various quality dimensions from these instruments and either use
a single item to measure overall satisfaction with an information system (Rai et al.
2002) or use a semantic differential scale (Seddon and Yip 1992).

The researcher believes that these alternative approaches highlights that UIS and
EUCS are not consistent in their roles as measures of information systems effectiveness as demonstrated by EUCS having outperformed UIS in the context of accounting
information systems. How then do UIS and EUCS perform in other verticals in assessing information systems effectiveness, and, if an inappropriate instrument is used
for analysis (for example, UIS for accounting system evaluation), how then does that
affect the resulting analytical results? How would this then impact on business decisions? The researcher also believes that the items stated which make up both UIS
and EUCS instruments (see above) constitute functional components of the instrument. Hence the information system it is measuring is viewed from a functional,
not strategic view, thereby supporting the argument that UIS and EUCS have little
relationship with the business goals of the firm.

Saarinen (1996) looks at this situation of evaluation of information systems effectiveness from a different perspective and introduces the consideration of cost/benefit
analysis as a more comprehensive and direct assessment of information systems

development projects. Cost-benefit analysis is essentially a comparison between two states. Proposed new system costs and benefits are usually compared with those of current systems whether they should be manual, partly computerised or fully computerised (Lincoln 1986). Post-audits of established systems however do not have such an obvious basis for comparison and it is essential to decide what the comparator will be before undertaking a study.

Saarinen (1996) extends the measure of success to include the development process (standing for the investment costs and efficient use of the resources) and the impact of the information systems on the organisation (standing for the benefits of the investment). Saarinen (1996) undertook a study to assess four dimensions of success—the development process, use process, information systems product quality, and impact of the information systems on the organisation, that he put forward as a means of measuring information systems success. These four dimensions were derived from his definition of a successful information systems development project, which is "The system development process leads to a high quality information systems product whose use has a positive impact on the organisation" (Saarinen 1996, p. 106).

The traditional investment analysis techniques and criteria, such as return on investment, net present value, or payback period are seldom used because of the unique nature of information systems investments (Saarinen 1996). This has led to evaluation criteria being supplemented by subjective judgment and surrogate measures such as UIS. Furthermore, information systems investments share many features with research and development investments, often having corporate-wide, intangible and long lasting effects. Therefore, economic evaluation and quantitative measures tend to be difficult to obtain and easy to manipulate. These measures seldom suffice in practice, but should be supplemented with subjective judgment and multiple diversified criteria (Cerveny and Clark 1985).

Subjective judgment and ease of manipulation of these measures cited by these authors raises the points of correctness and personal bias. For example, Saarinen (1996, p. 104), by asking the following questions, puts some perspective of the existing inadequacies of approach to information systems effectiveness measurement. He asks "How is then the result or outcome, in a case of an information systems investment, be characterised? Is it the information systems product itself or the net benefit of using it, or both? Furthermore, for whom should that result be favourable or satisfactory—the developers, the users of the information systems, or the managers?" Developers may aim at a high quality information systems product at minimum cost. User satisfaction may be determined by ease of use of the information systems and proper support for their own work. Managers, in turn, may prefer economic and quantitative values of both costs and benefits, giving an opportunity to compare the information systems investments with the alternative uses of these resources (Saarinen 1996).

The investigation (Saarinen 1996) was based on treating success as a four dimensional construct, consisting of the success of the development process, success of the use process, quality of the information systems product, and impact of the information systems on the organisation (Fig. 2.4). The two extensions (inclusion

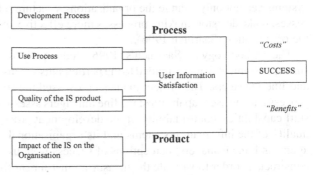

Fig. 2.4 Main Dimensions of Information Systems Success. (Adapted from Saarinen 1996)

of the development process and impact of the information systems on the organisation) align the subjective success evaluation better with the traditional cost–benefit paradigm, thereby increasing its content validity significantly (Saarinen 1996).

Success of the development process: Successful development of an information system requires capable and motivated users and systems analysts, who can effectively communicate and specify requirements for the system. The systems analysts must be able to design a system meeting these requirements, and to implement it into a technically feasible solution. They must also be able to help the users with the implementation process. All this has to be done to budget and time constraints. Measurement of the success of the development process can be based on an external view of the adherence to the given budget and time schedule (Lucas 1981). The success of the development process may also be measured with an internal view of the project, evaluating the level of developer and user expertise for the development exercise (Bailey and Pearson 1983).

Success of the use process: Evaluation of the use process can be done by the outcomes of the information systems services provided to the users; these should ensure that the information systems staff has those attributes and capabilities that would help them to communicate effectively and specify the users' needs. The information systems staff should be able to respond to the users' requests without undue delay (Saarinen 1996).

Quality of information systems product: Measurement of the information systems product quality is often based on the user perceptions of different attributes of the system. High quality information systems products should have both high system quality and high information quality (DeLone and McLean 1992). It should provide users with relevant and reliable information in the desired format. High system quality requires a good user interface and flexibility to allow for adaptation and expansion for the future.

Impact of the information systems on the organisation: The impact on the organisation of the information systems should be positive. The changes are measured in quantitative and monetary terms. Because these data are often difficult to obtain, surrogate measures, such as the manager's perceptions of change pertaining to such changes that affect the profitability of the organisation may be used. Information systems can not only change the organisations structure but also improve work processes, make decision-making processes more effective and intensify the controls of the organisation (Saarinen 1996).

The methodology for Saarinen's (1996) study involved the development of a measuring instrument that was mailed to the participants—consisting of project managers and line managers. The project managers assessed the success of the development process and the user capabilities; the line managers assessed the information systems staff capabilities, controllability of the development process and results, that is, the quality of the information systems and its organisational impact. The project managers' and line managers' perceptions of success were used for the first three initial constructs in order to validate the measuring instrument (Saarinen 1996).

Additionally, a modified version of the short-form UIS (Baroudi and Orlikowski 1988; Ives et al. 1983) was used in the study as a criterion for all four constructs. Seven-point scales where only the extreme points of the scales were labeled were used to score the data. The data was taken from the 200 largest companies and 25 of the largest banks in Finland. Altogether 272 information systems managers from these organisations were contacted. The response rate was approximately 50%.

The results of the study showed that of the four factors used to assess the impact dimension, decision-making and control, efficiency and profitability, use and change, and communication and restructuring, profitability was found to be related to the impact on the work processes and consequent cost savings. Saarinen (1996) in his concluding remarks makes the point that there are no generally acceptable measures available to quantitatively and objectively assess information systems success. The reliability of measuring instruments has been increased by the use of multi-item questionnaires. Saarinen (1996) also states that further research in this area needs to be undertaken.

Saarinen's (1996) study has been an attempt to extend the scope of UIS, which includes only indirect measures of success—the use process and quality of the information systems product—while his instrument measures success directly by success of the development process (standing for the investment costs and efficient use of resources) and the impact of information systems on the organisation (standing for the benefits of the investment).

Saarinen's (1996) model may be a step forward in establishing a more realistic and standardised means of measuring information systems effectiveness in that he concluded profitability was found to be related to impact on the work processes with consequent cost savings. Perhaps here one could introduce the possibility that this model represents a closer relationship with the business goals of the firm because it considers improved work processes while reducing costs. This would be likely to improve the overall efficiency of the firm, and enhance its competitive position in the market, surely the primary business goal of any firm. That being said, Saarinen (1996) includes UIS as part of his model, in spite of the fact that it has widely recognised shortcomings as an indicator of information systems effectiveness. There also seems to be a lack of a mechanism for the absolute definition of business goals for SISP in this model as with most other models. The varying views and controversy surrounding methodologies for assessing the evaluation criteria for information systems effectiveness measurement, as discussed, warrant the establishment by researchers and practitioners alike of a standardised approach to the process of evaluation of potential criteria for information systems effectiveness, to find and agree on a standardised approach. One early attempt at this was the SESAME model, as described in the following section.

2.3 Systems Effectiveness Study and Management Endorsement (SESAME)

A more standardised approach to cost–benefit analysis was discussed by Lincoln (1986). A large, consistent base of information was gathered using a standard methodology called Systems Effectiveness Study and Management Endorsement (SESAME) from a large number of applications across a range of industries. Previous analyses of barriers to IT use in the 1970s (Lincoln 1976, 1980) led to the establishment of a long-term program termed SESAME designed to explore computer investment appraisal issues. Using this base of information allowed senior executives to compare the financial performance of computer systems with other investments, to set reasonable financial targets for new systems development and to judge the 'return on investment' from their computer systems with that achieved by other companies.

Despite the wide use of cost-benefit forecasting to justify proposed system investments, executives remain skeptical about the level of benefits actually achieved. This is partly explained by the inherent uncertainties in the cost–benefit forecasting process. User reluctance to commit to future savings, previous large cost overruns, arbitrary estimates of system life, risk and inflation rates all erodes the credibility of any forecast. All too frequently, there is a lack of financial disciplines applied to the system development process—it is often unclear who is accountable for the benefit achievement and it is rare to find an information systems plan integrated with the business plans, and the user benefits are frequently described as 'intangible' and rarely post-audited (Lincoln 1986). Measurement of the business value of IT and factors that contribute to the success of information systems have been the subject of considerable research over the last two decades, and yet there is no single, widely accepted framework that could be employed in measuring impact of investments on IT (Davern and Kauffman 2000).

A report sponsored by the UK Department of Trade and Industry (Department of Trade and Industry 1984) reviewing the barriers and opportunities associated with information technology concluded that the main barriers to further use of information technology are the lack of appropriate cost–benefit techniques and the need to consolidate previous investments. This conclusion is a further example of the lack of a suitable framework for measuring the impact of investments on IT. Nothing much has changed over 20 years. For many organisations, measuring the outcomes of technology investments is a frustrating exercise because of the confusion over what should be measured and how to define the value of IT (Seddon et al. 2002; Tallon et al.

2000). The impact of information systems investment on performance also depends on contextual variables, such as the external environment, the organisational context and information systems maturity (Choe 2003). Kivijarvi and Saarinen (1995), Ragowsky et al. (1996) and Li and Ye (1999) have empirically shown the moderating effect of environmental uncertainty and the moderating effect of information systems maturity on the relationship between information systems investment and improved financial performance.

Business investments are judged to have value only if their contribution to the output of the business could be distinctly quantified (Sugumaran and Arogyaswamy 2004). The ability to assign value to IT business outputs is far more difficult than a simple cost–benefit analysis. Most IT investment decisions based on standard return on investment (ROI) and net present value (NPV) assumes a static scenario. These traditional measures of value often lead to inadequate or outdated IT systems. The debate is still continuing regarding what are appropriate independent and dependent variables to consider while assessing the effectiveness of IT with respect to productivity and performance (Sugumaran and Arogyaswamy 2004). This view has prompted Sugumaran and Arogyaswamy (2004) to propose a three-stage model linking environment/organisation to the value centre and to performance measures to provide conceptual guidance to select the most appropriate measure(s) of IT performance. They have recognised the fact that IT performance measures need to be tailored to fit with the purpose of the IT in question, and that the purpose itself is determined by external/internal variables.

An alternative means of evaluation of the impact of an information system change is a comparison of the same organisation before and after the system was introduced. The question being asked is then "Has the system brought an improvement in overall financial performance?" In many of the cases in the UK Trade and Industry study, this approach was found to be unsatisfactory due to changing environmental factors (Lincoln 1986). External environmental factors remain an issue in more recent time (Choe 2003). Other means of evaluation involve comparison against an alternative system. There are two fundamental questions to be answered with this approach; the first involves the basis for comparison and the options include the previous computer system, alternative technology or manual systems. The second concerns the level of service that will be assumed and the options range from the same level of service provided by the current system to not undertaking the activity at all (Lincoln 1986).

Not all computer systems lend themselves to this type of analysis. Strategic systems are usually so interlinked with business decisions that to dissociate the two becomes virtually impossible. Lincoln's (1986) experience has shown that after reviewing the options and thinking through the implications, most senior executives require an initial analysis against an essentially manual alternative system with a level of service that could be expected from a manual system. This raises the possibility that many executives still query whether the use of computer technology is beneficial even after many years of computer usage. As IT expenditures increase as a proportion of total expenditures, management is under constant pressure to justify the investment in IT and produce tangible evidence of this return on investment (Sugumaran and Arogyaswamy 2004; Petter et al. 2008; Miller and Doyle 2001). This also relates to another barrier or resistance to change pertaining to information systems effectiveness and integration discussed by Gation (1994) when she talks about personal agendas, bias and manipulation or misinterpretation of data. This facet of the planning and effectiveness measurement process is something that cannot be modeled out and will always be an unknown quantity. The recognition of multi-stakeholder perspectives adds further complications, raising issues such as power asymmetry, politically driven changes, technology-led changes and conflict objectives (Connell and Young 2007).

The SESAME project, by way of its design approach, laid the groundwork for a standardised means of assessing the value of information systems investment. It is timely at this point to examine the practical performance of SESAME in business and to ascertain the full impact it has had on IT project valuation.

2.3.1 Application of SESAME

Clearly, a consistent approach was required by Lincoln (1976, 1980) to alleviate the shortcomings of existing methodologies. The use of a consistent approach across a large number of applications also provides the capability of developing a statistical base. The SESAME approach has now evolved into a co-ordinated attempt to build a database of proven financial returns gained from the use of information technology. A SESAME study focuses on systems that have been implemented for at least twelve months and identifies in considerable detail the full costs and benefits experienced to date (Lincoln 1980). Once these are established, projections are made over the expected system life to a maximum of five years. The approach adopted by an individual study is tailored to specific requirements. When a before and after comparison is valid, it will be undertaken. In most cases of SESAME analysis, however, the approach has been a comparison against an alternative system.

SESAME is essentially a bottom-up approach, based on individual case studies, in contrast to top-down studies of the business impact of information technology (Cron and Sobal 1983; Strassman 1984; Yap and Walsham 1986). SESAME does not attempt to evaluate the full implications of a computer system. There may well be social and organisational implications for example, which a full and detailed evaluation would wish to consider. These social, environmental and organisational issues have been studied by Choe (2003), Kivijarvi and Saarinen (1995), Ragowsky et al. 1996, Li and Ye (1999) and Sugumaran and Arogyaswamy (2004) in recognition of the growing importance of these issues in consideration of planning and evaluative processes. SESAME set out to explore one dimension of the evaluative process in the hope that the results themselves would be of interest and would add to a fuller appreciation of the impact of computing on organisations.

The SESAME approach made three significant points in trying to understand the evaluative process for information systems development, implementation and impact. The first is the bottom-up approach based on case studies, which concurs with other authors, for instance Grover and Segars' (2005) work on rational—informal process in planning, creativity focus and wide participation profiles. The second is the recognition that the cost–benefit component of information systems effectiveness measurement is only one component of the evaluation of the full implications of the information systems. SESAME recognised that there are other influencing factors that exist and pose significant difficulties in assessing implications (Hirscheim and Smithson 1986). The third is that the SESAME program is tailored to the specific requirements of each individual study. This important feature illustrates that the SESAME program has the ability to recognise and allow for the nuisances of individual businesses. This facility is explored in more detail by Sugumaran and Arogyaswamy (2004, p. 85), who state "our primary intent has been to alert the user to the need to tailor IT performance measures to fit with the purpose of the IT in question".

Lincoln (1986) made the point that analyses of this type (SESAME) have proved to be valuable for senior management. The analyses enabled management to feel confident about financial returns available from technology and thereby allow a more rational investment policy to be developed. Equally, such analyses enabled senior management to remove the applications that are not financially viable and thereby enhance the overall return on investment made from technology. Another advantage of a standardised methodology such as SESAME is to use the results obtained to enable targets to be set for new developments.

Now the opportunity arises to establish a standard for effectiveness of applications in terms of return on investment, and the facility to undertake post-audits of the financial returns of the computer systems exists. Lincoln (1986) also suggested that all major computer applications should have clear cost-benefit targets established as part of the planning process and should be automatically post-audited. As information systems developed and expanded in general use, other issues and potential means of assessment of effectiveness have arisen, and these will be discussed in the following section.

2.4 Other Approaches to Information Systems Effectiveness Measurement

There are other approaches to the measurement of information systems effectiveness. Singh (1993), in his paper on using IT effectively, comments on IT and computer-based information systems (CBIS) being major concerns to the firm. This relates to firm performance, which is used as a measure of information systems effectiveness. In spite of the enormous potential of IT and CBIS, actual experiences of organisations have been less than satisfactory. Lyytinen (1987, p. 5) summarises these concerns as follows: "The information systems community faces a paradox: despite impressive advances in technology, problems are more abundant than solutions; organisations experience rising costs instead of cost reduction, information systems misuse and rejection are more frequent than acceptance and use." Organisations vary in their capacity to absorb IT and identify two important determinants being motivation and the ability to exploit IT.

Motivation is a function of the perceived value of IT to the firm in furthering organisational goals and objectives (Singh 1993). The survival and growth of both the firm and key individuals in the firm depends on results, which are measurable and quantifiable. Positive results motivate key individuals to experiment with new approaches and technologies. Ability creation has structural, procedural and behavioral dimensions. The relevant socio-technical skills have to be imparted to the concerned personnel; appropriate structural mechanisms must be put in place and a climate supportive of the use of IT must be created (Singh 1993; Klecun and Cornford 2005; Rondeau et al. 2006).

Furthermore, it is reasonable to presume that organisations will be motivated to change their planning processes over time in an attempt to improve their effectiveness as well as leverage their investment in information systems (SISP; Grover and Segars 2005). Firms are aggressively searching for new ways to leverage information, knowledge and IT in supporting strategic goals and competitiveness. Hence, SISP in many firms refers to both a proactive search for competitive and value-adding opportunities, as well as development of broad policies and procedures for integrating, coordinating, controlling and implementing the IT resource (Grover and Segars 2005).

A major concern to management practitioners and academics is to help organisations realize, in practice, the growing potential of IT/information systems. This is compounded and confused by the lack of a universal cohesive approach to SISP and information systems effectiveness measurement. Existing models may be characterized as growth stage, planning, project management or composite depending on their primary concern (Grover et al. 1996; Wang and Tai 2003; Henderson et al. 1987). The growth stage model is based on the premise that the process of the organization's adaptation and use of IT/information systems is an evolutionary one involving organisational learning and should therefore proceed through identifiable stages (Nolan 1979).

Planning models are directed towards producing an action blueprint to help an organization harness IT for enhancing its information/knowledge management capability and are functional at two levels—strategic and operational. After analyzing major planning models, Boynton and Zmud (1987) concluded that IT planning must be viewed as a continual series of incremental efforts to first surface and then resolve or exploit business problems and opportunities. These authors also hold the view that future projects in which the aim is to better understand the planning process are likely to be more significant than projects focusing on identifying additional issues to be addressed in the planning process. As planning evolves, companies are expected to realize that formal structures can make planning processes more efficient. Experience in dealing with uncertain technological options can yield more comprehensive decision processes (Grover and Segars 2005).

Operational level planning models tend to be much closer to information systems project management whilst strategic planning models vary considerably in their focus, scope and use (Singh 1993; Grover and Segars 2005). Project management models are used for developing tactical and operational level plans and schedules to facilitate effective implementation of IT/information system projects. These are based on traditional network methodologies, taking into account the peculiarities of information systems related activities, such as the level of risk associated with the project, project size, the degree of structure of the tasks to be automated and the level of technology of the project relative to the organization (Davis and Olson 1984). An integration of these planning model components makes a composite planning model possible.

2.4.1 Composite Planning Models

Composite planning models exist at strategic, tactical and operational levels in an integrated fashion. Evidence of increasing recognition of these models and their use is increasing in the literature (Singh 1993; Grover and Segars 2005; Petter et al. 2008). Historically firms' performances have been deemed sub-optimal due to shortcomings in the planning processes mentioned, being the highly fragmented nature of, and the narrowly focused approach to, the information systems planning and management effort.

While the limited domain of application of growth stage, strategic planning and project planning models is self-evident, prevalent composite planning models tend to provide a cursory treatment to implementation aspects. Many models are not context-independent as may be assumed, they have grown in a specific organization and invariably many changes have to be undertaken before they can be adopted for other organisations (Singh 1993). Lack of pragmatic orientation is evident in most models. Organisations have to make information systems related decisions in the "here and now" situation characterized by their history, the present context and the rapidly changing internal as well as external environments. Most models by themselves are of little help in deciding how to get started, how to adjust the plans to incorporate the latest technological advances, what organisational changes to make, when to abandon a system and a host of other questions (Singh 1993).

However, several useful trends were emerging. The scope of planning models was being continuously broadened, as was evidenced by an increasing number of comprehensive information systems planning models that incorporate strategic, tactical and operational levels. Importantly, integration and service quality was also being made an integral part of most comprehensive models (Petter et al. 2008). Most models also made provision for an external feedback loop (technology, competition, manpower) to help review and keep the plans current (Singh 1993). As organisations become technologically and geographically complex, the importance of planning activities increases. Accordingly, a planning culture often emerges in the form of highly structured systems. Rationality may be built into strategic planning systems through comprehensiveness (Fredrickson 1984; Sambamurthy et al. 1993), higher levels of formalization (Lederer and Sethi 1988), a focus on control (Boynton and Zmud 1987) and top down flow.

In spite of this continued research into planning, the literature seems to highlight a common fault in the planning process—something that one would think elementary, the identification of the core business competencies and business goals, and their alignment with IT planning. Ensuring then that alignment between business and information systems departments is paramount and rigorously enforced, the planning, development and implementation processes can take place. Singh's (1993) mention of an external feedback loop is essential for the continued success of the SISP and IT development, and is essential in helping to maintain the competitive advantage obtained by the information systems implementation by furthering the organisational goals and objectives of the firm. The feedback loop enables rescheduling of activities and redeployment of resources and facilitates monitoring and controlling tasks (Singh 1993). The planning system then should contain design characteristics that will alert managers to changing organisational and environmental conditions that may require a change in strategy (Grover and Segars 2005).

Another useful development in the early 1990s was increasing automation in the planning process that helped reduce the replanning effort and render feasible planning on a continuous basis. The increasing involvement of managers and top management in the planning and management of information systems functions was another adjunct to success in information systems use for the firm. The use of the firms performance as an indicator of information systems effectiveness, in view of the lack of a comprehensive and cohesive approach to information systems planning and a recognition in the literature that IT/information systems use and investment have been largely sub-optimal, is self-defeating. If the firm cannot plan for an outcome, how can that outcome be used as an indicator of success? Evaluation and analysis of planning models and what they should include continues today.

In their recent review of models, dimensions, measures and interrelationships pertaining to measuring information systems success, Petter et al. (2008) acknowledge that there have been substantial strides forward towards understanding the nature of information systems success. They give the example of the widely cited DeLone and McLean model of information systems success (1992) was updated a decade later based on a review of the empirical and conceptual literature on information systems success that was published during this period (DeLone and McLean 2003). Some researchers have synthesized the literature by examining one or more of the relationships in the DeLone and McLean information systems success model using the quantitative method of meta-analysis (Mahmood et al. 2001; Bokhari 2005; Sabherwal et al. 2006) to develop a better understanding of success. Others have started to develop standardized measures that can be used to evaluate the various dimensions of information systems success as specified by DeLone and McLean (for instance, Sedera et al. 2004).

While research has provided strong support for many of the proposed interrelationships among success dimensions in the DeLone and McLean model, more research is needed to explore the relationships that have not been adequately studied. Empirical research is also needed to establish the strength of interrelationships across different contextual boundaries (Petter et al. 2008). The Petter et al. (2008) qualitative literature review, in which 180 academic papers between 1992 and 2007 with some aspect of information systems success were reviewed, takes the first step by parsing out the results based on individual *vs.* organisational units of analysis. The study found that there is insufficient empirical evidence to evaluate most of the relationships at the organisational level. However, there could be other, more complex effects that could explain the relationship between these success constructs at either the individual or organisational levels of analysis. Petter et al. (2008) suggest that researchers may want to consider complex functions, such as curvilinear effects, that affect the relationships among information systems success constructs.

Researchers have also suggested that service quality be added to the DeLone and McLean model. An instrument from the marketing literature, SERVQUAL, has become salient within the information systems success literature within the past decade. SERVQUAL measures the service quality of IT departments as opposed to IT applications, by measuring and comparing user expectations and their perceptions of the IT department, and is discussed in the following section.

2.5   SERVQUAL as an Investigative Tool

Research by Parasuraman et al. (1985) concluded that service quality is founded on a comparison between what the customer feels should be offered and what is provided. Subsequent work by Parasuraman (1988) saw the evolution of the SERVQUAL scale for the measurement of customer perceptions of service quality. Parasuraman has reassessed and improved the scale during the following decade (Parasuraman 1991, 1993, 1994). There is support for this argument in the information systems literature. Conrath and Mignen (1990) report that the second most important factor of user satisfaction, after general quality of service, is the match between the users' expectations and actual information systems service. Rushinek and Rushinek (1986) conclude that fulfilled user expectations have a strong effect on overall satisfaction. The prime determinants of expected service quality, as suggested by Zeithaml et al. (1993), are word-of-mouth communications, personal needs, past experiences and communications by the service provider to the user.

A frequent contributor to the finished system's inability to meet the user expectations is the misinterpretation of user needs by the information systems department. A study by Laudon and Laudon (1991) reveals the failure rate to be between 35 and 75 %. The information systems department's communications influence expectations, in particular, the information systems can be a very powerful shaper of expectations during system development. Users are reliant on the information systems staff to convert their needs into a system. In the process, the information systems staff creates an expectation as to what the finished system will do and how it will appear. Laudon and Laudon (1991) found that all too frequently the information systems staff misinterprets user requirements or give users the wrong impression of the outcome because many systems fail to meet user expectations.

The notion that information systems departments are service providers is not well established in the information systems literature. As stated earlier in this review, six measures of information systems success have been identified (Delone and McLean 1992); Pitt et al. (2001) have augmented this list to include service quality. They used the instrument SERVQUAL to assess service quality as a measure of information systems effectiveness. Since system quality and information quality precede other measures of information systems success, existing measures are strongly product focused. This is not surprising given that many studies providing the empirical basis for this categorization are based on data from the early 1980s, when information systems was still in the mainframe era. The quality of the information systems department's service, as perceived by users, is a key indicator of information systems success (Moad 1989). User satisfaction is used by information systems departments to improve their quality of service provided (Conrath and Mignen 1990). The product supplied by the information systems department, a computer with software, is tangible. The intangible attributes associated with this product need to be considered in the context of information systems effectiveness measurement. That is to say, users/clients do not want just the machine, they want and possibly expect installation assistance, product knowledge, software training and support and online help. Current information systems success measures, product and system quality, focus on the tangible.

Pitt et al. (2001) argue that service quality, which is intangible, needs to be considered as an additional measure of information systems success. The results of their study led Pitt et al. (2001) to conclude that information systems service quality is an antecedent of use and user satisfaction. SERVQUAL has been validated as a suitable instrument to measure information systems service quality after examination of content validity, reliability, convergent validity, nomological validity and discriminant validity. Instruments such as SERVQUAL may be used as a diagnostic tool to measure information systems service quality (measurement of service quality prior to and after IS service quality change).

Pitt et al. (1995) evaluated the instrument from an information systems perspective and suggested that the construct of service quality be added to the DeLone and McLean model. The Pitt et al. (2001) study also assessed information systems effectiveness in different types of organisations using an investigative instrument. The study focused on service quality as a measure of information systems effectiveness. The role of the information systems department within the organization has broadened considerably over the last decade. Once primarily a developer and operator of information systems, the information systems department now has a much broader role. They have expanded their roles from product developers to become service providers (Pitt et al. 2001).

The introduction of personal computers results in more users of IT interacting with the information systems department more often. Users expect the information systems department to assist them with a myriad of tasks, such as hardware and software selection, installation, problem resolution, connection to local area networks, system development and software education (Pitt et al. 2001; Moad 1989). Facilities such as the information centre and the help desk reflect this enhanced responsibility. Information systems departments now provide a wide range of services to their users and have expanded their roles from product producers and operations managers to become service providers. The information systems department has always had some service component to its role, but service rarely appears in the vocabulary of the traditional systems development life cycle.

DeLone and McLean (2003) added service quality to their updated model, acknowledging that "the changes in the role of information systems over the last decade argue for a separate variable—the 'service quality' dimension" (p. 18). In recognition of other developments in information systems and related topics, other researchers have modified the DeLone and McLean model to evaluate specific applications such as knowledge management (Jennex and Olfman 2002; Kulkarni et al. 2006; Wu and Wang 2006) and e-commerce (Molla and Licker 2001; DeLone and McLean 2004; Zhu and Kraemer 2005). When applying the DeLone and McLean model to different practical applications, Petter et al. (2008) make the point that the DeLone and McLean model is naturally dependent on the organisational context, and that the researcher wanting to apply the DeLone and McLean model must have an understanding of the information system and organization under study. This will determine the types of measures used for each success dimension. The selection of success dimensions and specific metrics depend on the nature and purpose of the system(s) being evaluated. For example, an e-commerce application would have some similar success measures and some different success measures compared to an enterprise application. Both systems would measure information accuracy, while only the e-commerce system would measure personalization of information (Petter et al. 2008).

In their conclusion, Petter et al. (2008) recognize that measuring information success or performance in empirical studies has seen little improvement over the last decade. Researchers and practitioners still tend to focus on single dimensions of information systems success and therefore do not get a clear picture of the impacts of their systems and methods. They add that progress in measuring the individual success dimensions has also been slow. The work of Sedera et al. (2004) in developing measures for success is encouraging and this type of work should be continued in future research. Valid and reliable measures have yet to be developed and consistently applied for system quality, information quality, use and net benefits (Petter et al. 2008).

In a similar manner to the research and development of planning models, methods of information systems effectiveness measurement are the subject of continued research. Many researchers until the early 1990s (DeLone and McLean 1992; Ein-Dor and Segev 1978; Weill and Olson 1989) have noted the multi-faceted nature of information systems effectiveness rendering the use of a single overall indicator of information systems effectiveness unlikely. UIS is still popular as a single measure of information systems effectiveness but it is difficult to justify this as a comprehensive or adequate measure.

In their closing comments on this part of their review, Grover et al. (1996) make the observation that there are other studies that have utilised multiple criteria for information systems evaluation, these studies tend to be more comprehensive and able to alleviate the problem of limiting the amount of variance. These studies hypothesise how the variables related to one another and show promise. This approach however may be limited if the multi-criteria are in conflict. More recent work suggests that the use of UIS as a measure of information systems effectiveness is still being questioned. Gation's (1994) study looked at the relationship between user satisfaction and user performance for a particular system. Although her study overall supported the validity of UIS as a measure of information systems effectiveness, Gation raises the question of focused and relevant question selection for survey instrument in studies of this nature, and the possibility of careless or biased interpretation of results. DeLone and McLean (2008) revisited user satisfaction measurement. They considered the most widely used measures, those being the Doll et al. (1994) End-User Computing Support instrument and the Ives et al. (1983) UIS. They report a study by Seddon and Yip (1992) which found that the EUCS instrument outperformed the UIS instrument in the context of accounting information systems. The Seddon and Yip (1992) study also found that both the EUCS and the UIS contain items related to system quality, information quality and service quality, rather than only measuring overall user satisfaction with the system. Because of this, some researchers have chosen to parse out the various quality dimensions from these two instruments and either use a single time to measure overall satisfaction with an information system (Rai et al. 2002), or use a semantic differential scale (Seddon and Yip 1992). Others have used scales for attitude that are comparable with the concept of user satisfaction (Coombs et al. 2001).

Hackney and Kawalek (1999) believe that end-user involvement and business-IT alignment are important means to ensure information systems effectiveness—this view was ratified by Rondeau et al. (2006) in their study into information systems management effectiveness and end-user computing and its impact on manufacturing firms. Gerwin and Kolodny (1999) considered the role of an organisational approach to information systems planning on the basis that cross-functional decision pro cess creates greater work system integration and hence more information systems effectiveness.

Composite planning models, then, are continuously being evaluated and expanded as a result of extensive research in information systems planning and as a result of the expansion of information systems into other functionalities as technology advances. Areas such as knowledge management and e-commerce involving internet systems are now included in the information systems planning literature and in practical business. The discussion resulting from the volume of research being undertaken in information systems planning models is an indication of the complexity of the issue and the differing views on what is required for improved efficiency of planning models in the future. A consistent major inadequacy though, is what measure of information systems effectiveness should be used to assess the success of the planning process. This matter is also undergoing continuous and vigorous research in an effort to facilitate a standard approach to information systems effectiveness measurement, which would surely be a considerable positive advancement for the assessment of information systems planning. An evaluation of other methods of information systems effectiveness measurement follows in the next section.

2.5.1   Evaluation Perspective of Other Approaches to Information Systems Effectiveness Measurement

Individual level of analysis has been the dominant evaluative perspective, consistent with the popularity of perceived criteria and usage measures. Few studies deal with the perspective of external entities perhaps because researchers have examined effectiveness from within the organisational context, which is relevant, when information systems research focuses on data, information, or a decision. When information systems research focuses on information systems strategic impact, this approach is not appropriate. Hamilton and Chervany (1981) hold the view that multiple viewpoints should be incorporated into the assessment of system effectiveness. This may facilitate increased awareness of the value of information systems and to understand the multidimensionality of information systems effectiveness. This view was later explored from differing approaches by Hackney and Kawalek (1999), Gerwin and Kolodny (1999) and Rondeau et al. (2006). Hackney and Kawalek (1999) make the point that misalignments in information systems strategies, goals, and objectives may be avoided by increasing end-user involvement in planning. Gerwin and Kolodny (1999) comment on the dimension of cross-functional decision process and their implementation, which creates greater work integration and collapses traditional organisational boundaries. Rondeau et al. (2006) look at greater organisational involvement and the resultant revision of information systems management practices that better fit the information systems requirements.

Grover et al. (1996) make the point that improving information systems effectiveness is generally the goal of information systems research, that application of the results should lead to information systems effectiveness or success. The application of a myriad of IT in business process change and electronic commerce makes evaluation of investments even more important and complex. The construct model developed by Grover et al. (1996) is an attempt to provide a common set of dimensions for the evaluation of information systems effectiveness and there use in future studies will enable the acceptance of a common paradigm. Rondeau et al. (2006) developed a framework for assessing information systems performance which related organisational involvement in information systems development, information systems management effectiveness, end-user self-reliance in application development, end-user dependence on information systems expertise, and information systems performance and tested the framework in a survey of manufacturing managers. Their study concluded that increased information systems strategic planning effectiveness, more responsive and better designed computing solutions and more useful end-user training programs were significant improvements resulting from organisational cooperation and respect. The degree to which medical pathology practices, both private and hospital based, are able to coordinate such frameworks for information systems development and assessment will need to be investigated in the context of a contributing factor to information systems development success. The knowledge of such frameworks will also be determined. These issues will be further examined in Chap. 3 in which the literature pertaining to medical pathology practice is examined.

Grover et al.'s (1996) study also importantly recognizes the significance of more focus on impact evaluation and the organisational level of analysis due to the changing orientation of the field. Their study does so without distracting from the relevance of process or response evaluation. Rather the study calls for more attention to matching the appropriate type of evaluation with the unit of analysis, evaluative perspective domain of study, frame of reference and purpose of evaluation. This approach is also recommended by Petter et al. (2008).

Jiang et al. (2002) take a different approach and look at the process of information systems planning and information systems effectiveness in terms of the project team structure and relationship of its members as an adjunct to success. Projects are a major process structure for accomplishing many tasks in organisations (Peters 1999). A project is a non-routine, complex, one-time effort limited by budget, resources, time and performance specifications designed to meet customer needs (Gray and Larson 2000). In spite of obvious challenges this form of organization is used widely because historically it has been successful in the development of new software and hardware projects while satisfying customer requirements. The project team and the project manager are the two crucial components to implementing projects (Campbell 2005). Each component must be effective to promote the chances of project success (Schwalbe 2000). However, a variety of views in the project team may lead to conflict in tasks and personalities. The project manager may be powerless to remove any conflicts due to lack of authority over team members. Thus, building a cohesive, motivated project team is a key to ultimate accomplishment of project goals and the project manager has the primary responsibility for providing leadership to meet these goals (Peters and Homer 1996; Chan and Reich 2007).

It is obvious that effectiveness of both project managers and the project team is essential for the success of the project. Unfortunately, this effectiveness is hard to achieve and is even harder to define because of the different perceptions of system success between information systems staff team members and owner/user team members (Linberg 1999; Chan and Reich 2007). For example, the information systems staff team members may declare a project outcome successful if the system abides by information systems standards and policies for data security, accuracy, documentation and hardware and software compatibility (Jiang and Klein 1999).

By the same token, information systems users may consider the project outcome in terms of content and currency of information, the extent of the changes to their workloads and impacts on their jobs (Delone and McLean 1992). These differing viewpoints can lead to conflict. This conflict, if present in medical pathology practice, may represent a barrier to information systems planning success, and is a significant issue that requires evaluation by this research. Pre-project partnering, a collection of practices aimed at controlling conflict and system quality, have been proposed as a method for avoiding problems associated with multiple interests within a project (Larson 1997).

Pre-planning partnering involves a considerable up-front investment in time and resources to establish a foundation for teamwork during the project's duration. This involves institutionalizing procedures and provisions for continued commitment to teamwork, resolving disputes, attaining top management support and agreed upon

approaches for collaborative problem solving. The purpose of pre-planning partnering is to lay the groundwork for a successful partnering process (Jiang et al. 2002).
Under ideal conditions, pre-project partners should be selected from those who have
established a successful track record of partnering on previous projects. When this
is not possible, other strategies should be used. For example, Larson (1997) reports
that pre-project activities normally focus on getting top management's commitment
to the partnering process. This should involve an initial top management conference
that sets the tone for the partnership process and establishes the dialog to control
conflicting tasks and issues among those involved with the project.

Building a collaborative relationship between the major players is imperative. The
project manager for each partner has a major role in this by facilitating the breakdown
of barriers to collaboration and establishing trust and respect amongst team members
(Larson et al. 1992; Jiang et al. 2002). The team members bond through the development of a common set of goals and objectives, a process that reduces potential
conflicts. Pre-planning partnering also expands the commitment to other key individual members who will be working on the project, and may involve outside consultants,
well-versed in team-building skills facilitating a workshop on ice-breaking activities,
principles of teamwork, synergy and approaches to continuous improvement.

A study was undertaken by Jiang et al. (2002) to investigate pre-project partnering
with two research questions in mind. The research questions were—Do pre-project
partnering activities influence information systems project manager performance?
and Do pre-project partnering activities influence effective project team characteristics? The research methodology involved questionnaires being sent to randomly
selected members of the Project Management Institute (PMI). The membership is
widely used in other project management research, yielding comparability across
studies (Larson 1997). The items concerning pre-planning partnering investigated
were: before the project began people met to build a collaborative relationship; before the project began key people met to identify potential conflict areas; before
the project began documented processes were in place for joint resolution of problems; before the project began a formal charter stating shared objectives was drawn
up; the project included provisions for continuous improvement. Analysis of their
data supported the following hypotheses—pre-project partnering activities lead to
improved project manager performance; pre-planning partnering activities lead to
more effective team characteristics; strong project manager performance improves
effective project team characteristics; strong project manager performance improves
project outcomes and strong project team effectiveness improves project outcomes.

In their conclusion, Jiang et al. (2002) make the point that the implications of
their study are clear. Pre-planning partnering should be implemented to promote a
collaborative framework for conflict avoidance and resolution, and continual quality
improvement. The impact of this on the successful outcome of information systems
projects can only be positive and contribute towards more effectiveness in information
systems planning and development. The work of Jiang et al. (2002) is significant with
respect to business-IT alignment in SISP generally and could be adopted as a set
process for this undertaking. It would seem that the principle of conflict resolution in
their work is critical in improving the communication, co-operation and collaboration

between business and information systems staff in view of this widely recognised misalignment, which is discussed further in the following section.

2.6   Business-IT Alignment

Alignment between business and IT is inherently of value and contributes to organisational success (Chan and Reich 2007). The Society for Information Management conducts an annual survey to gauge the importance of various IT issues. In 2005, the number one management concern of all groups of respondents was alignment. Alignment was also ranked as the top management concern in 2004 and 2003. For two decades, IT alignment has consistently appeared as a top concern for IT practitioners and company executives (Luftman et al. 2005). For many years researchers have been drawn to the importance of business-IT alignment (McLean and Soden 1977; Henderson and Sifonis 1988). Chen and Reich (2007) have undertaken a review of the literature on this important topic with the view to ascertain where and how the research and business communities regard alignment. This research seeks to examine the literature on business-IT alignment relative to medical pathology practice, both hospital based and private practice, to ascertain how SISP is regarded by the medical pathology industry. Chapter 3 contains this examination, and from the content of the literature the researcher will formulate an approach for further investigation of this important contributor to SISP as applied to medical pathology practice.

Early research showed a number of approaches to achieving alignment—linking the business plan with the IT plan; ensuring congruence between business strategy and IT strategy; and examination of the fit between business needs and information systems priorities. Motivation for this early research on alignment emerged from a focus on strategic business planning and long-range IT planning in the early 1980s (e.g. IBM 1981). From a business perspective, planning was characterized as a top-down and a bottom-up process, and departmental (e.g. IT) plans were created in support of corporate strategies. From an IT perspective, decisions on hardware and software had such long-term implications that tying them to current and future plans of the organisational unit was a practical necessity (Chan and Reich 2007).

The business and IT performance implications of the alignment have been demonstrated empirically and through case studies during the last decade (Chan et al. 1997; de Leede et al. 2002; Irani 2002; Kearns and Lederer 2003). These authors' findings support the hypothesis that those organisations that successfully align their business strategy with their IT strategy will outperform those that do not. Alignment leads to more focused and strategic use of IT which in turn leads to increased performance (Chan et al. 2006).

There are a number of issues that require acknowledgement with respect to alignment mechanisms or models. The literature (Choe 2003; Wang and Tai 2003; Chan and Reich 2007; Rondeau et al. 2006) implies that there should be a priority between business and IT. That is to say that, whilst effective alignment of the IT plan with the business plan can provide competitive advantage, the opposite—aligning the business plan with the IT strategy—can result in potential losses. For this reason, researchers and practitioners should be cautious about putting IT in the lead (Kearns and Lederer 2000). Levy (2000) raises the issue that IT—even aligned IT—in and of itself is not strategic. In order for IT to be strategic, it must be valuable, unique and difficult for competitors to imitate. These two issues may in part explain why the outcomes of the implementation of enterprise systems in business are very often sub-optimal.

Chan and Reich (2007) discuss a number of challenges in attaining alignment, the first being those related to knowledge. These knowledge challenges refer to the central problem that IT executives are not always privy to corporate strategy, and that organisational leaders are not always knowledgeable about IT. Also, managers are not always knowledgeable about key business and industry drivers. One would perhaps then ask how did these managers attain their positions? It would be pertinent to suggest that if Jiang et al.'s (2002) ideas on pre-planning partnering and project team structure were in place, then the knowledge issue would not exist and alignment outcomes would be more favorable. It is also an interesting observation that in today's technology dependent and rich business environment there is now more corporate requirement for managers to have a basic IT qualification in addition to business qualifications.

The second challenge to alignment according to previous alignment research is the recurring issue that often corporate strategy is unknown (Reich and Benbasat 2000), or if known, is unclear and/or difficult to adapt. This poses a significant challenge because most alignment models presuppose an existing business strategy to which an IT organization can align itself. This would also make SISP difficult at best, impossible at worst, because there could be no business goals on which to plan SISP.

The third challenge to alignment is a lack of awareness or belief in the importance of alignment. Henderson and Venkatraman (1993) found that managers were more comfortable with business positioning choices than with IT positioning choices. This situation, as with the knowledge challenge above, could be alleviated by an approach to co-operative planning based on Jiang et al.'s (2002) research. Careful selection of people with the knowledge and attitude for team building and ensuring co-operation makes a positive impact on alignment and planning outcomes. Baets' (1996) research in the banking industry supports this approach. Baets (1996) found that IT alignment was hindered by a lack of knowledge of the banking industry amongst banking managers. Chan and Reich (2007) comment in the implications for alignment research that a number of issues need to be addressed. These issues which are shared responsibility for alignment; shared knowledge; building the right culture and informal structures; educating and equipping; embracing change; and focusing on essentials; are not only necessary to ensure improved business IT alignment but are equally necessary to ensure successful SISP and information systems effectiveness measurement. The incorporation of established and significant research such as Jiang et al. (2002) should be incorporated into any effort to make alignment and SISP more standardized and successful. Relating to some of these issues is information systems service quality, and this was recognised as an important consideration for the assessed success of information systems projects (DeLone and McLean 2003).

   The preceding sections have examined information systems planning approaches, principally business-IT alignment and pre-planning partnering, and information systems effectiveness measurement, which now includes service quality. In spite of a large body of research into these practices, there remain a number of issues that are dealt with in the following section.

2.7   Comments on Information Systems Planning Approach and Information Systems Effectiveness Measurement

The research on the approach to measurement of information systems effectiveness shows a great variation in the measurement techniques and the possibility of inefficiencies in the deployment of effectiveness measures through personal agendas or bias in the management team. Several authors, such as Pyburn (1983), Earl (1993), Sullivan (1985) and Sabhewal and King (1995) on SISP, agree that the planning process is most successful when rational and adaptive pathways are used in the design process. However, there is no mechanism suggested for possible pathways for this to happen, or overall consensus that this is the case.

   There are several other shortcomings in the planning models presented in business—lack of business-IT alignment; lack of consideration for team member selection in either top- down or bottom-up situations; lack of consideration as to how people communicate to make plans, that is knowledge management/extraction and organisational learning; lack of a clear definition of business goals by thorough business analysis involving stakeholders from management to end-users; and ensuring that the current information systems hardware/software has the capability to handle the planned information systems changes. The relativity of these cited issues to medical pathology practice, in particular laboratory information system capability, will be examined in the course of this research, and the structure of the planning process will be investigated through the emerging hypotheses.

2.8   Summary of Literature Review—The Broad Context

An extensive review of the literature pertaining to SISP and information systems effectiveness measurement has been undertaken. The literature review has revealed a number of components of the strategic planning and effectiveness measurement processes that are deemed by the authors cited as having high significance with respect to successful outcomes for the strategic planning and effectiveness measurement processes. These components were found to be end-user involvement in the planning process, business–IT alignment, pre-planning partnering and the recognition that the setting of an achievable business goal for SISP is an important strategic measure of information systems effectiveness.

   The more recent literature is drawing the attention of researchers and practitioners alike to emerging socio-technical and environmental changes that are taking place.

Petter et al. (2008) state that DeLone and McLean (2003) have modified their model to accommodate service quality as a result of a changing social emphasis. Information systems service is also recognised as a component of the function of an IT department. Petter et al. (2008) revisit the contention that practical application of the DeLone and McLean model (rightly) depends on the organisational context, but now that context has been broadened to include knowledge management and e-commerce. They also allude to the fact that as more research into information systems planning and success measuring is undertaken the other, more complex effects need to be considered when investigating items such as individual and organisational levels of analysis. Choe's (2003) work introduces a view that contextual variables, such as external environmental factors, have a moderating effect on information systems investment and improved financial performance. Chan and Reich (2007), in their review of IT alignment, found that challenges remain for IT alignment; they suggest more research be undertaken to investigate the process of alignment, contingency perspectives of alignment, measuring alignment and sharing knowledge.

There were other possible components of the strategic planning process, cost–benefit analysis, and information systems effectiveness measurement using UIS, that attracted considerable debate as to their true value in their respective roles, and are generally not seen as adequate measures of information systems effectiveness or information systems success by researchers. Cost benefit analysis is seen as functional and not strategic and takes no role in business–IT alignment (Choe 2003). The researcher takes the view that UIS is not a sound basis for the evaluation of information systems effectiveness. The researcher's view is that UIS should be part of the system design and subject to alpha and beta testing for approval by end-users before incorporating into the system that is to be implemented.

The discussion in the first part of the literature review has provided a well-documented basis on which the researcher can more forward into the area of research focus, that is, the medical pathology laboratory. The key argument of this literature review is that for SISP to occur, a number of components need to be in place, these being business–IT alignment, pre-planning partnering, and end-user involvement in the planning process, as stated above. There needs to be an objective and pre-planned means of assessing the success and effectiveness of SISP, and it is the researcher's view that this is the business goal(s) that is (are) driving SISP. That is to say, the measure of information systems effectiveness is the objectively measurable achievement of the pre-determined business goal for which the SISP was undertaken.

Chapter 3
SISP and IS Effectiveness Measurement—Pathology Practice

3.1 Introduction

The extensive search of literature into SISP and information systems effectiveness measurement reported in Chap. 2 revealed little work pertaining to pathology practice. What is recognised is that there is a task/technology asynchrony that is compromising laboratory information system performance in pathology practice (Brender and McNair 1996; Wells et al 1996). It is this gap that is the focus of this study. The modern pathology laboratory is a complex, heterogeneous environment, typically with a mix of autonomous and partially inter-working applications running on a range of hardware platforms. A consequence is that bigger pathology laboratories today (all main private pathology companies in Australia, for instance) are entirely dependent on their laboratory information systems functionality, and that the pathology laboratory information systems must be considered as 24 h mission critical systems (Brender and McNair 1996). Rapid evolution of laboratory procedures, methodologies and equipment characterises the pathology laboratory.

At present, the development of pathology laboratory science is so rapid that a vendor organisation has difficulty in absorbing, digesting and practically incorporating new enabling technologies/techniques into their version of a global laboratory information system. At one hospital site studied by Wells et al. (1996), an in-house pathology laboratory information system using object-orientated software tools based on a conventional file-sharing platform was found to give poor performance under load. Major investments have been made in IT/IS in pathology laboratories, which cannot be ignored. Hence, it is necessary that a pathology information system solution is future viable and able to incorporate already installed laboratory information systems functionalities. Therefore, an obvious laboratory information systems solution for the pathology laboratory domain is a solution based on a concept of open interconnected systems, interoperating on a functional level (Brender and McNair 1996). An example of an open systems architecture and design philosophy is given in the following section.

M. Belkin et al., *Strategic ICT Planning in Pathology*,
Healthcare Delivery in the Information Age,
DOI 10.1007/978-1-4614-4478-7_3, © Springer Science+Business Media, LLC 2013

3.2   The Establishment of the OpenLabs Project

The establishment of an open architecture implies that a market will develop for modular, scalable and cost-effective pathology information systems features without the dependence on individual manufacturers and hardware/software platforms which characterises current systems (Brender and McNair 1996). With this in mind, a consortium was formed in 1991 as part of the European Community's Advanced Informatics in Medicine Programme and included partners from industry, academic institutions and hospital laboratory services.

In 1992, the OpenLabs project began work with several major objectives: to improve the efficiency and effectiveness of pathology information systems by integrating knowledge-based systems with pathology information systems and equipment; to provide and implement standard solutions for electronic data interchange between laboratories and other medical systems; to specify an open architecture for an integrated pathology information systems; and to demonstrate the integration of various knowledge-based system modules on the open architecture platform and with existing pathology information systems (Boran et al. 1996).

The OpenLabs project is an ideal example to cite as an objectively planned and implemented SISP because the project involved all the concept factors suggested in the literature in Chap. 2—empowerment, motivation, innovation, pre-planning partnering, co-operative planning, information systems use, UIS and working towards a business goal. The OpenLabs project has taken as its core problem the definition of a computing infrastructure in which existing pathology information systems are accommodated and in which new functions or modules can be easily added. The main elements of the OpenLabs solution comprise a set of advanced laboratory services, a communication architecture including a coding system, generic interfaces to existing legacy systems, and a service manager to co-ordinate the overall computing environment (Boran et al. 1996).

The OpenLabs project services, in principle, any number of services providing support to the different aspects of a clinical laboratory which could be incorporated into the OpenLabs computing environment. The prototype service modules of the OpenLabs solution include: support for requesting laboratory investigations; automatic re-scheduling of additional investigations; performing laboratory investigations (advanced laboratory workstations); interpreting laboratory results; telematics for remote requesting and reporting; and managing the laboratory's use of resources by simulation (O'Moore et al. 1994).

In a trial at a major hospital in the United Kingdom, the ordering of pathology services by clinicians was aided by the use of knowledge-based systems. The ordering system automatically recommends pathology investigations appropriate to each patient's clinical condition and recent pathology. The doctors review the recommended tests and add to, delete from or simply accept the tests proposed for the patient. Routine use has resulted in a significant reduction in the number of tests ordered, a significant saving in medical staff time and improved appropriateness and continuity of management (Boran et al. 1996).

Another OpenLabs service is the advanced instrument workstation service, which was designed and developed on the basis of user requirements assembled from 13 partners with a range of complementary pathology laboratory expertise within the OpenLabs project. The gathered information was the result of discussions, local questionnaires, interviews, experiences and market analysis by industry partners (O'Moore et al. 1994; Boran et al. 1996).

The OpenLabs business process represents an intensive, objective and thorough SISP, but it is not referred to as such by the consortium—perhaps this is an industry nuance. It is in stark contrast to most other literature and studies cited in this review, and it is argued that the OpenLabs project represents a better approach to SISP. The OpenLabs project embraced several of the cited contributors to successful SISP (for example, end-user involvement, business–IT alignment and pre-planning partnering) cohesively in the same project. Many of the measures used by other authors (Doll et al. 1994; Ives et al. 1983) and recognised as a means for measuring information systems effectiveness, such as information systems use, user information satisfaction (UIS), decision-making and system quality are used by the OpenLabs team as requirements for the design process. The sole criterion for measurement of the effectiveness of the OpenLabs project is its ability to meet the design brief, which was stated as the definition of a computing infrastructure in which existing laboratory information systems are accommodated and in which new functions and modules can easily be added. The UK project met this goal and therefore can be considered to be successful and effective.

3.3 Achievements of the OpenLabs Project

The OpenLabs communications architecture had to achieve two important goals, firstly, the provision of an environment for facilitating the integration of modules implementing the advanced OpenLabs services, and secondly, the provision of an open solution by which these modules could be developed with a vendor-independent approach, that is, provide portability and interoperability in a heterogeneous distributed computing environment. Furthermore, there was a need for the system to be configurable so that some or all of the advanced OpenLab services could be integrated whilst having the facility to customise their use to suit a particular laboratory.

Existing legacy systems to be integrated within the OpenLabs computing environment include clinical analysers and pathology information systems generic interfaces capable of being configured to a wide range of existing instruments. The OpenLabs service manager controls the information flow between different modules connected to the OpenLIS (the OpenLabs pathology laboratory information system), thereby supporting the workflow in the pathology laboratory and enabling the management of pathology laboratory production in a highly computerised domain. The use of the generic interface and of system editors enables a high degree of flexibility in the configuration of the system for individual user requirements—a key function for information systems effectiveness.

The OpenLabs system has been designed to assume an interactive role in the interpretation of some key clinical results. Through a structured evaluation methodology, the system can provide interpretive comments of routine results and is programmed to provide alarms if interpreting abnormal results in the acute and high-dependency hospital environment. This facility has been found to considerably improve the efficiency and turn-around time of the laboratory (Boran et al. 1996).

The project team has introduced an important component in the design and planning process with the realisation that any information system requires continual assessment and "fine-tuning" to maintain maximum impact on the firm. The OpenLabs open architecture approach is a major step forward for pathology laboratories in being able to break free of the restrictions of commonly used mainframe systems. The ability to embrace modern technology and improve efficiency and effectiveness within the pathology laboratory environment sets the agenda for improved business outcomes and the ability for the pathology laboratory information systems to grow with the business and with the rapidly increasing developments in modern technology.

The OpenLabs project and its impact on pathology laboratory computing is significant for this study as it has documented (Boran et al. 1996; O'Moore et al. 1994) what amounts to a successful SISP undertaking in a pathology laboratory environment. The OpenLabs project also makes the association of a planning exercise with business outcomes as a measure of information system effectiveness. The OpenLabs project has provided a link between SISP in general business and SISP in pathology practice for this research. The OpenLabs project has also provided some insight into what is achievable technically in pathology laboratory computing, and this will be expanded in the following section.

3.4   Future Directions for Pathology Laboratory Information Systems

Brender and McNair (1996) have proposed user requirements and future directions of pathology laboratory information systems in their paper on user requirements on future pathology laboratory information systems. They put forward the following as the main user needs and requirements for future IT solutions in pathology laboratories: IT solutions must be highly flexible and maximally customisable—by the users themselves; IT solutions are based on the concept of open systems, both technically and functionally, which enables modular functionalities from different vendors to co-operate in forming a global pathology information systems functionality; IT solutions are future viable and able to incorporate already installed IT functionalities; IT solutions support management of failure prevention, of repair, of success and of change. The authors conclude that the establishment of an open architecture implies that a market will develop for modular, scalable and cost-effective pathology laboratory information systems features without today's dependence on individual manufacturers and hardware/software platforms (Brender and McNair 1996).

The popularity of open architecture systems developed considerably with the advent and increasing use of client-server technology (Anandarajan and Arinze 1998). The two major contributing factors to the increasing use of client-server technology at that time were technical factors and economic factors (Anandarajan and Arinze 1998; Wells et al. 1996). The technical advancements in IT have converged to make client-server computing possible through faster and minimised hardware components, and open standards that have created portable, scalable and inter-operable systems. Software trends such as graphical user interfaces (GUI), fourth-generation programming language and the advent of component-ware has also helped in the evolution of client-server information systems (Anandarajan and Arinze 1998). The ability to perform processing on desktop workstations instead of mainframes has considerably lowered the cost of computing for many industries (Anandarajjan and Arinze 1998). The limiting factor to development and enhancement of pathology information systems with open architecture and client-server technologies is the presence and reliance of a current mainframe information systems (Anandarajan and Arinze 1998; Wells et al. 1996). The laboratories studied in this investigation currently use mainframe systems, and their ability and desire to change to these more modern technologies will be assessed in the course of this investigation.

3.5   Other Areas of Information Systems Development in Pathology Laboratories

Other areas of information systems/software involvement in pathology laboratories found in the literature include a study by Mayer (1998), in which he describes the use of a commercially available financial management package to perform a cost-benefit analysis in a hospital pathology laboratory. The results obtained by the cost-benefit analysis were a major factor in the decision-making process for the management and development of the laboratory. This research (Mayer 1998) demonstrates the all too common piecemeal approach to pathology laboratory management and the decision-making process in pathology laboratories, unsupported by effective information systems management tools and perhaps full and proper business analysis.

Economic constraints within the healthcare system advocate the introduction of tighter control of costs in pathology laboratories. Detailed cost information forms the basis for cost control and financial management. Based on cost information, proper decisions regarding priorities, procedure choices, personnel policies and investments can be made (Mayer 1998). The package studied by Mayer (LabCost) serves as a general management tool for resource handling, accounting, inventory management and billing. The study involved cost–benefit analysis to aid the decision-making process concerning the purchase of a new analyser. The increasing need of pathology laboratories to implement cost control is a direct consequence of the unprecedented pressure to improve the financial efficiency of the laboratories and to reduce their operational costs. Whilst cost analysis is being increasingly used in the pathology laboratory to support management decisions concerning financial alternatives, most pathology laboratory directors find it increasingly more difficult to deal with the complex financial issues of the pathology laboratory services (Kreig et al. 1978).

Mayer (1998) recognises that there are several shortcomings to the process of cost-benefit analysis: costs vary with pathology laboratory size, spectrum of services, volume of work and types of equipment. Therefore, it is not possible to compare costs occurring in different laboratories; different levels of cost analysis are required for different levels of management; cost evaluation is expensive; cost analysis is usually based on historical data—the validity therefore of past cost evaluation for prediction of future trends has to be regarded cautiously; and most importantly, the inability of cost analysis to evaluate the clinical usefulness of the tests in terms of financial benefits that result from the test performance.

In his concluding remarks, Mayer (1998, p. 61) argues that "Due to cost containment, pathology laboratory analysers can no longer be selected only on the basis of their quality and capacity". The fact that cost is seen as the sole determinant in equipment selection, usually by upper/senior management, is important. The laboratory then may be forced into a position where it cannot take advantage of any technological advancement that a new analyser may have because it is deemed to cost too much to run.

Mayer's (1998) work on cost-benefit analysis as a means of improving cost efficiency in pathology laboratories is significant in that it points out that consideration of costs as the sole determinant of efficiency improvement can negatively impact laboratory quality that may compromise patient well-being. The cost-benefit approach may also be viewed as a functional means of efficiency planning, and as such it is not strategic. There are several views on what contributes to strategy and the means by which they may be included in a planning exercise and these are examined in the following section.

3.6 Development of a Framework for SISP

In spite of suggested pathways for SISP (Pyburn 1983; Earl 1993; Sullivan 1985), no mechanism (model) has been proposed to demonstrate how SISP should be approached for application to pathology information systems. Grover and Segars (2005), in their evaluation of the evolution and maturing of SISP, found that many studies had focussed on planning content with particular interest in methods and measurement of alignment between business and information systems strategy. Grover and Segars (2005) also found that these studies did little to illuminate the organisational aspects of planning. Earl (1993) made the observation that SISP approaches based on a degree of rationality and adaptability built into the planning process seemed to be more effective. This was thought to lead to a more effective basis for managing increasingly diverse and dispersed technologies across the organisation (Boynton and Zmud 1987; Zmud et al. 1986; Lederer and Sethi 1998). It would seem from their research that an effective mechanism for SISP is yet to be determined.

An extensive search of the literature into SISP and information systems effectiveness measurement in pathology practice revealed little work in this specific area.

To hypothesise an effective mechanism for SISP, we can consider the approach adopted by the OpenLabs team. The approach used by the OpenLabs team was to utilise the components of SISP and the setting of a clearly defined business goal to be used as a measure of information systems effectiveness, in a cohesive and cooperative manner.

Through the formation of a consortium to discuss, plan and implement the system, the following concept factors were embraced—empowerment, motivation, innovation, pre-planning partnering, co-operative planning and team building, information systems use and UIS (end-user involvement) and most importantly working towards a business goal. A model for the OpenLabs project is represented in Fig. 3.1.

The most dramatic difference in the OpenLabs approach as opposed to other approaches cited is that the OpenLabs team had a clearly defined goal for SISP, that is—the establishment of a modular, scalable and cost-effective open architecture pathology information system without the dependence on individual manufacturers or vendors. The achievement of this goal is the sole measure of the effectiveness of SISP and the information system. The approach used in the OpenLabs project with a clearly defined business goal as the measure of SISP success and information systems effectiveness could set a direction or standard for SISP projects. This is because the OpenLabs project team recognised that such previously and inappropriately used measures of information systems effectiveness (information systems use and UIS) were regarded as part of the system design is another important step in the rationalisation of an effective mechanism for SISP.

Figure 3.1 represents the project structure from the pre-planning partnering stage through to completion and shows the components of SISP in the OpenLabs project. The planning stage has integrated team selection and building with a clear definition of technical requirements of the new system. The model also shows that the new system has to be scalable for the future and have a platform that will facilitate integration with future technologies. The model also shows the relationship between the single measure of information systems effectiveness and SISP success—that being the achievement of the previously defined business outcome.

There are however shortcomings with this model. There is no allowance for future change (business and economic as well as technical) and no allowance for maintenance of competitive advantage. The model is also static and uni-directional—it has a start and a finish. For any future changes to the information systems another SISP has to be undertaken. A further question remains: "What facility does this model have for monitoring the effect of internal and external influencing factors on the present and future degree of effectiveness of the information systems?"

Chapter 3 has served to highlight that there is a lack of knowledge of SISP in pathology laboratory settings. The measurement of information system effectiveness can be shown to link with business outcomes as per work by Boran et al. (1996) and O'Moore et al. (1994) on the OpenLabs project. In the investigator's opinion, these authors' approach to information effectiveness measurement represents a more accurate assessment of effectiveness than other methods discussed. The OpenLabs

Fig. 3.1 OpenLabs
SISP/information systems
effectiveness model

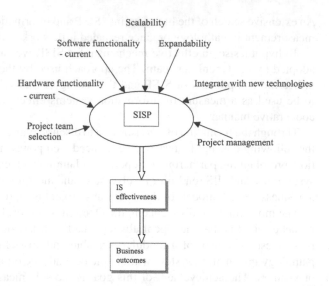

Fig. 3.1 OpenLabs SISP/information systems effectiveness model

project represents the only major strategically driven planning exercise in pathology laboratory computing that was found in the literature and it may be regarded as an important benchmark reference for this study. As well as investigating the components for successful SISP, such as business–IT alignment, end-user involvement and pre-planning partnering that are generally discussed on an individual basis when considering their impact on SISP; this study seeks to investigate the effects on SISP in pathology laboratory information systems when the components are considered to be acting together. This study will also investigate the role of the existing pathology laboratory information systems capability in the particular context of it being able to support strategic and technological change. The key issues stated here will help to demonstrate the shortcomings of the current pathology information systems capability, a lack of business-IT alignment and an inability for modern pathology laboratories to progress their businesses in parallel with other knowledge-based companies.

3.7   Key Issues of the Study

Stasis in technological development in pathology laboratories has existed for many years because of the persistence of mainframe pathology information systems. The systems use older, inflexible software not compatible with modern technologies (Brender and McNair 1996; Boran et al. 1996; Wells et al. 1996). There is little, or no, facility for the pathology laboratory to embrace web technology and all its ramifications. A web-based system would allow the pathology laboratory to utilise such facilities as wireless communications, web-based voice recognition software, telemedicine, and centralised supply chain management and human resource management (Brender and McNair 1996; Boran et al. 1996; Bossuyt et al. 2007). The ability to eliminate workplace boundaries, introduce a completely paperless laboratory, real-time communication between all interstate and overseas branch laboratories and introduce real-time standardised management facilities is non-existent (Bossuyt et al. 2007). The ability for a pathology practice to implement these technical and management facilities would represent a considerable strategic development, and should bring strategic pressure to bear on the practice(s) to undertake such change. The change would require SISP to be successful, but as noted above, the stasis of the existing mainframe information systems precludes SISP from occurring. The efficiency, effectiveness and profitability of the pathology laboratory are compromised considerably by this and the business outcomes are negatively impacted. With the international expansion of some of Australia's laboratories, this lack of modern technology integration ability must be detrimental to effective globalisation of the organisation and negatively impact SISP. Therefore the first key issue to be explored is that:

Lack of functionality of current laboratory information systems negatively impacts SISP effectiveness in medical pathology information systems.

It is common for senior management of pathology laboratories to use financial considerations in an attempt to increase profits (Friedberg 2008). The frequently used avenues available to senior managers are take-overs and mergers to attempt to take advantage of perceived benefits of economies of scale; negotiating with reagent/instrument suppliers for absolute minimum costs; and to keep reducing the labour cost component (Bossuyt et al. 2007; Mayer 1998). None of these financial measures used to reduce costs involve technology and full business analysis, and they are self-limiting (Choe 2003; Sugumaran and Arogyaswamy 2004). In the pathology laboratory this financial considerations approach provides information that forms the basis for evaluation of operations and decisions concerning the introduction or elimination of tests and services, choices of procedures, modification of methods and introduction or replacement of equipment (Mayer 1998; Klecun and Cornford 2005). These alternate measures are difficult to fit into a strategic plan both for the present and the future, and have little capacity to consider outside business and economic changes that may impact on the firm. The second key issue is that:

Decisions based on financial considerations negatively impact effective SISP in medical pathology information systems.

The literature refers to the bottom-up approach and the rational component in SISP (Petter et al. 2008; Earl 1993; Sabherwal and King 1995; Grover and Segars 2005). It also details a step-by-step method that this may be facilitated—empowerment → motivation → innovation → information system effectiveness. Involvement or empowerment of end-users in the design process leads to motivation and a feeling of ownership of the project—the end-users are enthusiastic to use the system and this assists with innovations to further enhance the project (Jaing et al. 2002; Hackney et al. 1999; Klecun and Cornford 2005). There is a lack of this involvement of end-users in the SISP in pathology and as a result a perception that the pathology laboratory information system is ineffective. The generalised negative attitude by end-users in pathology practice is attributable to the fact that end-users involve all staff from department heads and pathologists to junior scientists. The end-users involved in initial laboratory planning, both in information systems and workflow, are department heads and senior scientists. These staff members interact with senior management and the IT staff. The more junior scientists are engaged for their input that may have a more functional view as junior scientists attend to the physical testing of specimens and hence have greater use for the core functional processes of the laboratory information system. The third key issue for investigation is that:

Lack of involvement of end-users in SISP (specifically in pathology in Australia) negatively impacts on information systems effectiveness.

In pathology laboratories in Australia, there is a varying degree of business/IT alignment. Often the scientists are not involved in the planning or development processes of the pathology information systems at all (Brender and McNair 1996; Bossuyt et al. 2007). IT/IS service is lacking with respect to dissemination of information regarding changes or developments to the current system, and in-house training for end-users. The shortcomings of the current in-house systems frequently compromise changes and developments end-users may suggest because of inadequate technology to support these desired changes or developments (Boran et al. 1996; O'Moore et al. 1994; Connell and Young 2007; Friedberg 2008). The business/IT misalignment present in pathology laboratories, which contributes to the lack of empowerment and pre-planning partnering with end-users in the development process and the lack of facility of current systems to support many of the wants of the end-users (Friedberg 2008; Brender and McNair 1996; Boran et al. 1996; O'Moore et al. 1994) leads to decreased motivation and innovation (Jaing et al. 2002). This negatively impacts the role that the current laboratory information systems has in assisting the business to grow and increase its competitiveness in the market. This key issue will be investigated in the context of:

The greater the degree of business-IT alignment the more effective SISP is in medical pathology information systems.

There is little research undertaken pertaining to SISP and information systems effectiveness measurement in pathology practice throughout the world. The OpenLabs project (O'Moore et al. 1994; Boran et al. 1996; p. 75) represents an SISP exercise in pathology practice, but is not referred to as such by the participants in the project. There appears to be an ignorance of SISP and information systems effectiveness terminology in pathology practice. Little other research in strategic development of information systems in pathology laboratories is reported (Wells et al. 1996; Connell and Young 2007; Bossuyt et al. 2007; Friedberg 2008). The research relating to implementation and integration issues has resulted largely from a recognition by workers in pathology laboratories throughout the world that there are major problems with pathology laboratory IS in laboratories and there needs to be considerable changes made to rectify these problems (Friedberg 2008; Bossuyt et al. 2007; Brender and McNair 1996). Defining the problems facing pathology laboratories strategically is difficult without knowledge and experience in the components of SISP and a means of effectively measuring the outcome of an SISP exercise. In common with all things in life, knowledge is obtained from education and research. Therefore, an approach to change the use of standardised investigative tools and models is not suited to pathology laboratories at this stage because of the lack of research and education,

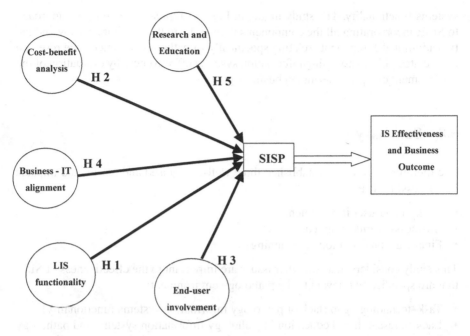

Fig. 3.2 The research model

and hence knowledge of SISP of the potential participants. This also negatively impacts pathology practice in terms of not having a standardised means to objectively investigate current problems and find an ordered solution to move forward. The fifth key issue for investigation is that:

Lack of laboratory information systems research and education negatively impacts SISP effectiveness in medical pathology information systems.

The relationships of the key issues are represented in Fig. 3.2.

The structural model shown in Fig. 3.2 is a representation of key issues developed from the literature review relating to successful SISP (end-user involvement in planning, business–IT alignment and cost–benefit analysis) and two additional items (pathology information systems functionality and research and education) investigated in this study with particular reference to pathology practice. Each individual item is initially assessed by a survey and quantitative analysis to investigate the relationships between each of the items in SISP in pathology laboratories. The structure of the model proposes that each item contributes to SISP. The model also proposes that any information system effectiveness measure embraces the achievement of a pre-determined business goal. The structure of the model also implies that all five items act in harmony, in a positive manner for SISP to be successful. Contributing factors to some items, such as pre-planning partnering (Jaing et al. 2002) are assessed in the context of end-user involvement to give added depth to the investigation. Assessment of a possible task-technology gap (or a reality gap, as Connell and Young (2007) refer to it) is undertaken in the investigation of pathology information systems functionality. The study model in Fig. 3.2 represents a cohesive approach to SISP, incorporating all the components derived from the literature review and the two additional components relating specifically to pathology practice. The research also relates SISP to assessing information systems effectiveness by evaluation of the achievement of a pre-determined business goal.

3.8 Summary

The literature review has established three well-recognised and researched impacts on successful SISP:

- Lack of end-user involvement
- Business–IT misalignment
- Financial considerations in planning

This study considers that two other issues are important to the effectiveness of SISP that are specifically relevant to the pathology environment:

- Task–technology gap (lack of pathology information systems functionality)
- Lack of research and education in pathology information systems and pathology laboratory management.

This study extends the conclusions of many of the authors cited in this chapter and the Chap. 2 about what contributes to both successful SISP and what are suitable measures of information systems effectiveness. The study model proposes a dependant relationship between them.

Chapter 4
Focus Groups 1 and 2: The Laboratory

4.1 Introduction

This Chapter outlines the first qualitative component of this research. It involves two focus groups (FG1 and FG2) conducted within the medical pathology industry. The aim of the focus groups is to evaluate the initial findings from the data analysis of the survey and assess their impact on the research question *"How does the effectiveness of laboratory information systems impact on business outcomes in medical pathology practice?"* A third qualitative component follows in Chap. 5; it involves a third focus group (FG3). Its aim is to discuss secondary findings from the quantitative data analysis and outcomes from FG1 and FG2 in a more theoretical sense. The outcomes of FG3 are then applied to the research question to elicit an overall picture of the research domain and its proposed implications for SISP in general, and pathology laboratories in particular. These outcomes are detailed in Chap. 6: discussion and conclusions.

Since assessment of the research propositions cannot be based solely on facts as it involves *values* such as SISP success, a means to consider the subjective feelings of participants was undertaken by way of focus group research. The focus groups were expected to provide information that the quantitative analysis was unable to (reflected in the percentage variance explained being < 100 %), by elucidation, analysis and understanding of respondent's feelings. "By the term qualitative research we mean any type of research that produces findings not arrived at by statistical procedures or other means of quantification" Strauss and Corbin (1998, p. 11). Morse (1991, p. 120) claims that qualitative research is appropriate if "(a) the concept is 'immature' due to a conspicuous lack of theory and previous research; (b) a notion that the available theory may be inaccurate, inappropriate, incorrect or biased; (c) a need exists to explore and describe the phenomenon and to develop theory; or (d) the nature of the phenomenon may not be suited to quantitative measure." A focus group would elucidate people's feelings about newly developed theories and variables from a quantitative analysis.

The FG1 and FG2 questions were framed around the five propositions derived from the literature review that were supported or not supported in context by the findings of the quantitative analysis of the data from the research instrument. The five

M. Belkin et al., *Strategic ICT Planning in Pathology,*
Healthcare Delivery in the Information Age
DOI 10.1007/978-1-4614-4478-7_4, © Springer Science+Business Media, LLC 2013

propositions are that lack of functionality of current laboratory information systems negatively impacts SISP effectiveness; cost–benefit (financial considerations) negatively impacts effective SISP; lack of involvement of end-users in SISP negatively impacts information systems effectiveness; the greater the degree of business–IT alignment the more effective SISP is and lack of laboratory information systems research negatively impacts SISP effectiveness in medical laboratories. Information from the participants of FG1 and FG2 was sought to expand on, and to seek explanation for the findings of the survey analysis, namely that financial considerations has no impact on SISP; that laboratory information systems functionality is the dominant proposition over business–IT alignment; and end-user involvement in SISP in pathology practice. The ramifications of laboratory information systems functionality being dominant in influencing SISP were particularly sought out as it could be the major hindrance to SISP and hence information systems effectiveness in pathology practice. These propositions would be the basis for the original theories derived from this research and pertaining to SISP and information systems effectiveness in medical pathology. FG1 and FG2 served to triangulate the findings of the quantitative analysis back into the general literature, thus validating the application of quantitative analysis to this project, and by laying the groundwork for future research to explore the theories evolved from this research. FG1 and FG2 would also themselves validate the research instrument questions used in the quantitative component.

As stated in Chap. 2, four laboratories were approached regarding conducting the focus group at their respective laboratories. Two declined to participate citing reasons of restricted time and staff shortages. The usual practice within research is to conduct focus groups and to have the participants off site from their working environment to eliminate distractions. In sympathy for the workload and staff constraints, the researcher decided there would be more chance of participation by laboratory staff under these circumstances if the focus group were conducted at the prospective participants' laboratories. The offer of a supplied lunch was made to help entice participation and to provide a more relaxed atmosphere to conduct the focus group. This occurred with FG1. FG2 was conducted after hours and off site at the request of the participants to allow for an uninterrupted discussion session.

4.2 FG1: The Hospital Laboratory

The focus group was conducted at a major public hospital laboratory. The focus group was conducted in the middle of the day, in a private room where the participants would not be disturbed or the focus group interrupted, and was attended by five participants (Table 4.1).

The researcher made sure, when negotiating with the laboratory manager, that the participants of the focus group were not the same staff who had completed the survey. This would then ensure that the focus group responses were spontaneous and unbiased.

Table 4.1 Focus group 1 participant details

Participant	Description and Qualifications
Participant 11	Principal scientist in microbiology and involved in middle management—*B.App.Sc*
Participant 12	Supervisor scientist in biochemistry—*B.App.Sc., PhD*
Participant 13	Supervisor scientist in biochemistry—*B.App.Sc.*
Participant 14	Supervisor scientist in haematology—*B.App.Sc.*
Participant 15	Senior scientist in haematology—*B.App.Sc.*

The role played by the researcher during the focus group discussion was one of observer. Additional notes to the focus group questions and responses were made by the researcher to promote further discussion and to help with the interpretation of the discussions and passed onto the facilitator to gain further understanding from the participants. The focus group was conducted by the researcher's senior supervisor, who acted as facilitator, and was assisted by the researcher's second supervisor. The focus group was recorded on two digital recording devices, one being a backup in case of a recorder failure. Before the commencement of the focus group, each participant was asked to complete an RMIT human research ethics form, which detailed that the project had ethics committee approval, and that the project was to be recorded and that the material could/would be published in this work and other academic journals and articles. The RMIT human ethics research form also explained that each participant was free to withdraw from the focus group at any time, should they wish to do so. It was stressed to the participants by the facilitator that anonymity and confidentiality were assured.

During introductory session, it was explained to the FG1 participants that the benefit of conducting a focus group was to investigate the relevance of the survey to the participants as laboratory practitioners. Surveys are answered not necessarily in the way we think because of the limited number of alternatives presented in the survey. The focus group can help investigate other possible alternatives to those presented in the survey. FG1 proceeded well with all participants actively contributing to the discussion. There was little prompting required by the moderator as the discussion, once a topic was determined, flowed freely.

The main issues to emerge from the first focus group discussion were:

1. There is a very low priority for funding for pathology, in particular for laboratory information systems development;
2. Pathology is held in poor regard by many other services in the hospital, especially the hospital management and some specialist departments;
3. There is no involvement of laboratory staff in development planning within the laboratory—especially with respect to the state government's Healthsmart project;
4. There is no research and formal education provided for laboratory information systems development, laboratory informatics and laboratory management; and

5. There is no co-operation between scientists, IT staff and hospital management
   in the development of laboratory services, which depend on the laboratory
   information systems.

Each of these issues is discussed in detail below.

4.3   Low Priority of Laboratory Information Systems

4.3.1   Management Considerations

The participants reported that there is very little consideration given by the hospital
management as to the needs/wants of pathology and therefore their allocation of
funds is minimal. The pathology department holds a low-priority level in the eyes of
hospital management, and other ancillary hospital/medical services. This situation
then leaves the laboratory short of staff and with no funds for basic development
of the laboratory information systems. The efficiency of the pathology department
is therefore further compromised, as the department is unable to update equipment,
principally the laboratory information systems, that would enable more efficient
and cost-effective workflow processes. This was illustrated by participant 13 who
commented—"*we would love to have a paperless laboratory, and be able to get
more management information but the current system cannot accommodate these
functions*".

The lack of cohesion between hospital management and the pathology department
is further illustrated with respect to discussion by the respondents about the hospital
steering committee concerned with the Healthsmart[1] system (a generic whole-of-
hospital information systems and initiated by the state government), and further
highlighted the laboratory's plight with comments suggesting that the hospital would
embrace this system without any consultation with the laboratory staff. Laboratory
staff feelings were negative to this as the staff had no idea what the system does
and how it would impact pathology; Participant 11 stating—"*we have been told we
are getting Healthsmart; we don't know what it does, we will just have to use it*".
The laboratory staff had not been involved in much discussion with the Healthsmart
steering committee. This was an issue of laboratory staff as end-users (as a component
of successful SISP), considering that they have no input into the planning process.

---

[1] Healthsmart is the Victorian government's whole-of-health information and communications
strategy for the public health sector. Healthsmart aims to improve patient care and reduce the ad-
ministrative burden and associated costs by adopting a more standardised approach to information
systems.

4.3.2   Financial Considerations

The participants in FG1 noted that lack of finance is the sole factor limiting the development of the laboratory, which requires a capable laboratory information system. Participant 11 commented—*"because they could get away with basic equipment if they can and turnaround times are not seen as a high priority, pathology has a low priority. There is a shortage of money in the whole network—a freeze on staff. There have been no new ideas for the last 4 years."*

The inability of the pathology department to improve the efficiency of the laboratory information systems is due principally to financial constraints that have led to a situation promoting over-ordering of tests. The participants also noted that some doctors, having not received the results on patients ordered the previous day, simply order the test again. This results in senior pathology staff members having to cross-check daily requests from hospital doctors to eliminate double ordering of tests. This issue was illustrated by Participant 12—*"this can take one hour, it can take two hours of your day as a senior person. The computer should be able to do this."* The problem then results in a cost escalation at the hospital that is twofold:

- Multiple duplicate test ordering, and
- Senior staff time cross-checking test requests.

The participants agreed that the allocation of funds for the public sector is a different process than that for private pathology and has different pressures/considerations for outcomes. Participant 11 elaborated—*"The amount of funding varies with which political party is in power at the time. Private pathology gets money from income and investment"*. The identity and hence priority held by pathology is also a consideration when the hospital was allocating funds. The participants believe that the image of pathology and scientists is poor and as a result, pathology has a low priority in the hierarchy of the hospital; for example, Participant 13 noted—*"I don't think there has ever been a high priority for pathology work in any public hospital over the years. It is not seen as a high incentive or priority for them to do anything. I have worked in a few public hospitals and it is always the same—pathology is always on the lower end of the scale with money and equipment—never seems a high priority."*

Participant 12 also remarked that—*"this image of low priority has meant little consideration is given to pathology when considering who gets what out of the overall hospital budget"*. The participants agreed that this scenario has been compounded in the past by a hospital CEO who was also insensitive to pathology department's needs. The fact that the clinical importance of pathology in the hospital is out of balance with the priority for provision of funding required to enable the turnaround times that would be commensurate with in-house critical medical situations was agreed by all participants. There is an enigma here—the laboratory has little priority for funding as it is not regarded as being an important or significant part of the medical/diagnostic team, and so is neglected financially—and yet its services are frequently required in a mission critical scenario to provide test results for critically ill patients.

4.4   Lack of Capability of Laboratory Information Systems

4.4.1   Communications—Impact on In-House and Peripheral Business

The participants agreed that there is a lack of capability in the laboratory information system at the hospital. The laboratory information systems lack of capability, they said, to facilitate commonly used communications technology, such as e-mail and broadband, is a severe strategic restriction as their laboratory is unable to compete in the market for local general practice referrals. Participant 13 stated the results of this situation—"*we have lost GP work simply because the laboratory information system cannot e-mail results*". The participants stressed that the lack of communications ability of the laboratory information systems also creates a significant and potentially compromising situation for in-patients in the hospitals' critical wards (Intensive Care Unit, Cardiac Care Unit). The participants gave an example where the laboratory receives specimens from patients in these critical wards and can perform the tests requested and have the results available before the patient's details can be entered on the laboratory information system. The current laboratory information system, the participants noted, does not allow for patient details to be entered in the ward. Participant 12 alluded to an impact of this shortcoming—" *the doctors are on the wards all day—being able to do electronic requests would help in the laboratory— something we are looking at and the state is looking at with Healthsmart.*" The outcome of this scenario, the participants said, is that the results therefore cannot be entered on the laboratory information systems and delivered to the ward. Participant 12 continued—"*This creates an unacceptable time delay for patients as there are complaints about this from the doctors and specialists in these wards. This delay may potentially compromise the patient*". The use of wireless technology has been trialled in some emergency departments in Melbourne and the idea to import this technology had been raised within the laboratory and, according to the participants, was impossible to pursue due to lack of capability and adaptability of the laboratory information systems. As has been noted by the participants, this situation would be difficult to change due to financial constraints on hardware purchases and the required software changes.

4.4.2   IT Support

The IT support to the pathology laboratory was acknowledged by the participants as consisting of two IT staff members, who assist scientific staff with basic computer maintenance but who cannot assist with any software development. Participant 13 described the situation by stating—"*IT is run by 2 people—that is grossly under resourced—they do PCs, cabling, software and look after the hardware—they do the whole works, and they know nothing about pathology.*" The Pathology Department is under resourced, the participants noted, with respect to simple hardware requirements such as replacement hard-drives and screens in the event of their failure—further evidence of poor funding.

A lack of disaster recovery/redundancy in the current laboratory information system was also highlighted by the participants, not only in the context of laboratory information systems lack of capability, but also in the context of more operational and basic functional issues, such as redundancy planning, back-ups and programmed obsolescence of hardware.

The participants agreed that as a consequence of the lack of IT support by staff that are knowledgeable of the laboratory information systems functionality, senior staff are at times involved in simple changes to the system such as test set layout. When this occurs it puts a strain on the other staff to cover the seniors in their absence. This negatively impacts the laboratory's turnaround time. Participant 11 added—*"There are no meetings between laboratory staff and IT staff to co-ordinate any laboratory information system changes and enhancements, or functional management changes—Melbourne Medical Centre pathology has never had a computer group to look after the laboratory information system or anything like that—like meetings on what we want to do and what we would like to have on the system—it is all ad-hoc really."*

4.4.3   Laboratory Management Tasks

The participants pointed out that the scientists are unable to perform simple management analysis processes such as workflow analysis, design of workflow systems and simple budget analysis. They noted that senior scientists have little access to any financial figures, and it takes a considerable time to find/extract any financial data from the laboratory information system. The participants acknowledged that the main thrust of "management" data provided by several laboratory information systems refers to patient numbers referred by each doctor and the number of different tests performed each day. Participant 14 remarked—*"we can get patient number data but it is always weeks in the past—it takes so long to get any information from our system"*.

The participants agreed that the ability of the laboratory to perform tasks, or provide information for the performance of tasks such as workstation analysis, workflow analysis and associated roster building and costing, benchmarking and reagent tracking in real time is nonexistent.

4.4.4   Paperless Laboratory

The participants raised the issue of a "paperless" laboratory as another example of how workflow and time are compromised by lack of capability and lack of changeability of the laboratory information system. Discussion with respect to an example ensued—the haematology analyser (an instrument that tests blood to provide data to help provide diagnoses) produces numerical and graphical data (22 parameters) on each patient sample analysed. The laboratory handles approximately 1,300 patients per day. The number of individual test results, as opposed to test set results (A full blood examination (FBE) = 1 test set and has 22 individual test results) for the department of haematology alone would be $1,300 \times 22 = 28,600$ individual results. These results are passed from the analyser to the laboratory information system to report stations in strings of the 22 result characters plus a unique patient identifying number and an episode number. The total number of characters for each patient having an FBE may be as high as 38. Time is lost in the finding, matching and stapling of request forms and data print outs. The participants pointed out that this also increases the risk of transcription errors, and has cost components for labour, paper and staples. The participants noted that most, if not all, haematology analysers today have a powerful PC to control the analyser—it would be possible to network these together through the mainframe, they suggested, to provide a paperless laboratory. Participant 14 elaborated—"*in haematology at the moment, we still actually staple the request to the analyser print out and look at every one of those FBEs and validate it. There are no validation rules in the computer—we have got rules in our heads.*"

The participants noted that validation rules could be used from the abnormal flags the analyser produces, thus providing the paperless laboratory which all participants agreed would be a major development in laboratory efficiency. As the participants had mentioned earlier, any development effort to accomplish this is not possible due to the geographical barrier having the software writer in Bangkok (see p. 219 for complete details), the laboratory information systems lack of capability and hospital cost constraints.

Examples of other technical problems with the laboratory information system were given by the participants, a significant one being that when individual test results from other departments are added to a patient file (the most common scenario is for multiple test sets to be ordered) then the amount of data packets that the laboratory information system has to deal with is quite considerable. Participant 13 made the point that "*when there is a lot of data going through the system, it just about stops. The file sharing mainframe has a real problem with lots of data*". The laboratory information system cannot accept the graphical information, they said, which is important for the scientist in interpreting haematology results, and so it has to be printed and attached to the doctor's request form. The participants noted that the doctor's request form is able to be digitally scanned into the laboratory information system but they pointed out that integration between the scanning software and the laboratory information system is sub-optimal involving several key strokes to change from one screen to another (it is not possible to visualise the image and the results at the same time on the system).

4.4.5   Laboratory Information Systems Research

The comments made by participants and the mood of FG1 portrayed a lack of co-operation and synergy between the management and the laboratory staff. The participants noted that there appears to be no cooperative group for providing direction in technological and service development in laboratory capability and strategy. It should be noted, despite the participants addressing issues surrounding the enhancement of their competitive position in the local pathology market, did they use the terms "strategy, business development, business–IT alignment and laboratory information system effectiveness". The participants noted that the main thrust of research in laboratory information systems centred on auto-validation of results and middleware.[2] Without middleware, they went on to explain, laboratories would not be able to use modern analysers and have them interfaced to the laboratory information system.

Middleware is a growing field of IT development, the participants added, presumably because laboratory scientists and IT staff consider the prospect of developing a laboratory information system that embraces "new" IT technology too difficult— particularly in terms of implementation in place of the existing laboratory information system, and too costly. The participants pointed out that there is, however, no customisation in middleware design—the middleware dictates how the laboratory must use it. As Participant 12 noted—*"the two main topics of investigation in medical scientist journals are auto-validation and middleware. Autovalidation is software that is specifically written to automatically validate test results, and it must consider matters such as multiple diseases, multiple drug regimes and their possible interactions, and multi-department test results"*. The hospital laboratory information system cannot integrate fully with the middleware, the participants added, and this compromises the middleware installation and functionality, as Participant 12 explained—*"middleware is a compromise anyway because it comes as a standard package and never suit individual requirements. Even with middleware the laboratory still has its work practices dictated by the software."*

4.5   Hurdles to Hospital Laboratory Information Systems Development

4.5.1   Software Development

The participants in FG1 noted that the lack of capability of the laboratory information system at the hospital is significantly further complicated by there being only one person who can develop and change the software and *"he lives in Bangkok"*. Participant 11 gave some background to the situation—*"it was written by this programmer guy—he was the team leader who wrote it. Gradually all the other users have stopped using it—he has taken the licence now."* A lack of awareness and understanding of the SISP planning process by scientists, IT staff and management in this hospital is

---

[2] Middleware is an intermediate software between a more technically advanced analyser and the current "old" generation of laboratory information systems that enables the analyser and the laboratory information system to integrate (Friedman 2005).

also a very considerable barrier to any attempts to develop the laboratory information system with a cohesive, planned and integrated method. The measurement of information system effectiveness is therefore also compromised in the hospital.

4.5.2   Vendor Laboratory Information Systems

It was noted by the participants that the prospect of working with the vendors to modify and customise a system for their laboratory was not attractive because it was expensive and very time consuming in terms of trying to get the vendors to make the changes. Participant 15 detailed some of his experiences with vendor software—*"the commercial systems are off the shelf software and do not exactly meet the demands of the laboratory. The use of this off the shelf software meant that the laboratory has to work around the software; that the vendor software does not fit the workflow processes of the laboratory thereby limiting the laboratory's functionality"*. Vendors often do not keep adequate records, the participants also noted, of which laboratory information system contains customised changes. The ramifications of this are that vendors would therefore not necessarily be familiar with any particular system. The alternative of building an in-house system was, to the participants, equally unattractive due to time and financial constraints. Again, it would seem from the participants' comments, that there is little or no chance that this laboratory could obtain a laboratory information system that entirely suits their needs—this fact is severely compromising the effectiveness of this hospital laboratory in providing adequate services to in-patients and out-patients alike, the participants added. It can be seen from analysis of the discussion in FG1 thus far that the hospital environment places the laboratory under pressure to perform from two perspectives:

1. A fast turn-around capability that must be viewed as "mission critical" for desperately ill patients in emergency, ICU and CCU.
2. The facility to compete in the market locally to attract referrals from local general practitioners; this facility must provide integration with the general practitioners wants with respect to turn-around time, report format and report medium.

4.5.3   Workflow Analysis as a Development Tool

With respect to "management" information and its application to the laboratory information system developmental process, the participants noted that the senior staff receive only quarterly cost centre and laboratory financial reports. The participants believe that it is complicated to retrieve any financial data from the laboratory information system. They went on to add that there are virtually no management data, such as test numbers per day, readily available with their current laboratory information systems; Participant 14 stating—*"with the current laboratory information systems, if people ask if the workload has increased or decreased, I would not have a clue—I can't get any stats."* The fact that this seriously compromises attempts at management/business planning by laboratory senior staff was made abundantly clear by the participants, Participant 14 adding—*"how can we plan when we don't have real time test numbers to plot and compare with last year so we can calculate growth?"*

They went on to illustrate the situation by example—if the laboratory information system is unable to supply data relating to workflow analysis and hence staff requirements/time (rosters), goal setting (meeting performance targets as an adjunct to rapid turn-around times), reagent tracking and supply chain management, best practice and benchmarking are not achievable.

4.6   Laboratory Information Systems Wish List

There was consensus amongst the participants that with enough people and money, they could make their existing systems satisfactorily functional. In the view of the participants, people and money resources would be better applied to building a totally new system that would allow the scientists to re-engineer the whole laboratory and review and improve every facet of its operation. The participants' arguments against a vendor-supplied system were based on their view that a vendor system lacks customisation, and the implementation time and expense in achieving such changes are excessive. These customisation changes would be necessary to tailor the system to the work practices of the laboratory, the participants stressed. In the opinion of the participants, a web-based laboratory information system was thought not to be beneficial and was thought to have doubtful advantage over the infrastructure of the system presently in situ. This was an interesting attitude given the lack of education and research into information systems and business/management development; the lack of such knowledge as strategic information systems planning (SISP) and information system effectiveness measurement. Also, it is interesting given the discussion on technology such as wireless portables that was supported by the participants earlier in FG1.

4.6.1   Summary

The key findings of FG1 which focused on pathology practice in a public hospital were:

1. The pathology department is regarded within the hospital structure with low priority, and therefore does not attract funds for laboratory development, which includes development of the laboratory information system. Political reasons contribute to the low priority with which pathology is regarded, both internal

Table 4.2 FG2 participants' details

Participant	Description and Qualifications
Participant 21	Principal scientist in biochemistry and involved in middle management—*B.App.Sc.*
Participant 22	Peripheral branch laboratory manager—*B.App.Sc.*
Participant 23	Senior general scientist—*B.App.Sc.*
Participant 24	Principal scientist in haematology—*B.App.Sc.*

hospital politics (i.e. the CEO's view of pathology in the hierarchy) and federal politics (i.e. the incumbent political party's policy on health spending).

2. End-users, from department heads to junior scientists, are not involved in planning processes.
3. There is a task-technology gap that has had a negative impact on business outcomes for the hospital laboratory.
4. There is no IT department support for basic routine processes such as back-ups, and disaster/redundancy planning. There is no IT department support for laboratory information system development.
5. There are no management data available to assist with the management and potential planning of the pathology department.
6. There are no special interest groups or forums for laboratory management or laboratory information systems.

In the next section, a focus group conducted in a private pathology context is described and analysed.

4.7   FG2: The Private Pathology Laboratory

FG2 was held after hours and off site from the participants' workplaces at the request of the participants so that the meeting could be conducted without interruption. All four participants have at least 20 years' experience in private pathology laboratories and all participants have worked in more than one private pathology laboratory. The details of the participants' qualifications and current positions are detailed in Table 4.2.

The participants were selected for their length of experience in private pathology in Melbourne, which for all participants, involved working at more than one practice. This gave the researcher access to the participants' views on several laboratory information systems. The researcher ensured that none of the participants had participated in the survey (Chap. 5). As with FG1, each participant was asked to sign consent to participate form, in keeping with the protocols set down by the RMIT university ethics committee. The participants were informed that the focus group was being recorded and that the material would be used in this work and for possible academic publications. The participants were also informed that they were able to withdraw from the discussion at any time if they wished to do so. The researcher introduced the focus group with a short dissertation on the benefits of conducting a focus group (see p. 3, Chap. 6), and the background to the research.

The focus group proceeded readily with active discussion from all participants. The main issues to emerge from the discussion of FG2 were similar to those main points that came from FG1. The main points from FG2, the private pathology laboratory were:

1. Co-operation between scientists, upper management and IT staff is virtually non-existent for the development of the laboratory information system;
2. Funding for laboratory development is based on minimal cost expenditure, and does not involve the laboratory information system;
3. There is no laboratory informatics or laboratory management courses available;
4. Conferences and the few papers that are published in medical science journals are concerned with middleware and not overt redevelopment of laboratory information system; and
5. The laboratory information system is not regarded as an important part of the laboratory business by the upper management in private pathology.

Each of these issues is discussed in detail below.

4.7.1   Management Considerations

The participants of FG2 agreed that the relationship between scientists and management with respect to laboratory information system planning is functionally non-existent. Management relates to the IT department staff, the participants noted, and works to develop additional functionality in the laboratory information system, but this functionality is directed towards report delivery and the accounts department. The participants pointed out that there is a void between management, scientists and the IT staff with respect to development—as Participant 22 noted *"management makes decisions without any consultation with us"*. The result of this has been seen by all four participants within the laboratories in which they have worked, Participant 23 commenting *"I remember several occasions where the IT guy would let us know about a change they had made—we had no formal training with the change (or the whole system for that matter) and we were expected to use it"*. Participant 21 added—*"often the change did not help us, some were a disadvantage. I remember in one laboratory where they told us we had to use a bar code scanner to get up a patient's file, but it would not read the bar code labels they had printed. When I said buy some proper labels, the reply was we were told by management to try and print them, as it is cheaper. The end result was we could not use the bar code reader"*.

Scientists' ideas and their input into the development of the laboratory information system, in the experience of the participants, have not been welcomed by management or the IT staff either in the past or currently. The participants added that in general, the scientists therefore feel that it is futile to try and become involved in any development of the laboratory information system in the current climate of non-cooperation. The participants expressed a view that the laboratory information system was not regarded by staff as generally having any importance, other than to generate results. As Participant 24 said—*"everyone thinks that it is there to send out reports. We can't do much else with the system and because of years of frustration, we don't try now"*.

4.7.2 Financial Considerations

The participants noted that laboratory spending in private pathology laboratories in Melbourne concentrates on the purchase of analysers for which the best reagent deals can be struck. This situation further illustrates the lack of acknowledgement that scientists receive from management, the participants added, and it may ultimately compromise cost effectiveness for the practice. Participant 24 gave an example of this—*"for years we had used brand A for our haematology analyser. The laboratory manager, as instructed by the CEO of the practice, informed me that we were to change to brand B, which I knew from my colleagues who were using it, had technical inadequacies. I had a meeting with the CEO to inform him of the problems we would have if he went ahead with brand B. He stated that he had signed a contract because the reagents were cheaper, and that was the sole driver for his decision, and that his decision was final. Within two years we had changed back to brand A because the inadequacies of brand B were costing us so much in checking results"*.

The researcher raised the question of why this attitude to spending within private practice exists. The management and IT staff do not have an informed view of the benefits of a properly integrated analyser—IT relationship, and the efficiency of the laboratory is suffering as a result. Participant 21 raised an interesting perspective that may explain many negative attitudes towards the laboratory information system by suggesting—*"we are talking around the system as if nobody wants to know about it, as if it isn't there—like a commodity"*. Being regarded in this manner by the laboratory staff generally, and the upper management staff in particular, would have a considerable bearing on the allocation of funds, the participants agreed. Participant 24 expressed—*"to change to a totally different platform, say a web-based system, would cost a fortune—and for what benefit?"* Spending, as has been observed by the participants, is therefore functional and not developmental. The researcher acknowledges that the view of commoditisation of the laboratory information systems and the type of spending acknowledged by the focus group warrants further discussion and investigation and will be put to the participants of FG3 (Chap. 7) for that purpose.

4.7.3 Lack of Capability of the Laboratory Information Systems

The participants acknowledged that the laboratory information system in private pathology is regarded as a closed system and lacks both adaptability and scalability.

All four participants have been through mergers between private practice laboratories and have seen large increases in workloads. The participants noted that the inadequacy of the laboratory information system in providing laboratory management details such as workstation analysis and test versus time graphics compromised the smooth transition between the participating laboratories of the mergers. As a result, they said, the merged entity lost a considerable amount of work because of the difficulties that arose in servicing referring doctors test requests. Participant 21 illustrated the problem—*"we merged with practice A, which was using a very old in-house system written in Cobol and running on a mainframe. It could only store results for three weeks, then they had to be microfiched. Within two weeks of the merger, because it took forever for us to find results for the doctors, we had lost twenty percent of the doctors referrals"*.

The participants reported that there are some serious shortcomings in the private laboratory information system with respect to adaptability and integration. Participant 22 commented—*"the systems can't adapt to the workflow, they are static. They are resistant to change—I think everyone thinks it is too hard to change them now"*. This raised some discussion by the participants on middleware, as was the case in FG1 in the hospital laboratory (Chap. 6, p. 201). The participants of FG2 pointed out that in the private laboratory also, analyser vendors are more frequently implementing middleware solutions to help cover the inadequacies of the current laboratory information system, in an effort to allow laboratories some access to the more modern technology and clinical advantages of their analysers. One of the major hindrances to integration of new technology analysers is the lack of a common interface, the participants added; each analyser has to have a specifically written interface to the current mainframe systems in use in private pathology. Participant 24 elaborated on this scenario—*"if we want a new high tech. analyser these days, more often than not we need an intermediate system because we can't interface the analyser to the mainframe—so we have PCs all over the place in the lab and barely enough bench space to do the work"*.

The participants went on to add that the only area of laboratory information system development in private practice pathology is the area of auto-validation, where a series of rules are written into the laboratory information system to facilitate validation of results without scientist or pathologist intervention. They said that this applies to biochemistry and haematology primarily. The question of cost effectiveness for this approach was raised, as the time, complexity and cost of developing such a system against the time and cost of maintaining validation with experienced scientist and pathologists could potentially be much greater.

4.7.4   End-User Involvement in Planning

In the experience of the participants of FG2 within the various laboratories in which they have worked, there is no evidence of a cohesive, group approach to laboratory information system planning. Changes are made to the laboratory information system at the behest of the IT staff, senior management or laboratory manager, as is the case with the auto-validation programs and they said the general staff remain uninformed and untrained on the changes. As participant 22 commented—*"we put ideas forward but no-one listens. We have always had to learn the systems as we go—there is no formal training"*. The participants also reported that as a result of the lack of formal training on the laboratory information system, the scientists are compromised in their knowledge of the full functionality of the system, to the detriment of efficiency.

The participants added that there is therefore a lack of ownership, which is known to create a negative attitude towards an information system amongst the users, further compromising laboratory efficiency (Singh 1993). Participant 24 mentioned *"years ago there used to be user group meeting, supported by vendors, to foster discussion on laboratory equipment and information system—that does not happen now unfortunately"*. Participant 23 mentioned that he had seen a few employment advertisements for scientists with an interest in laboratory information system to work with the vendors as "Application specialists" to assist with training and implementation of new technology and to foster co-operative development of laboratory information system. Participant 23 added—*"maybe the vendors are waking up to the fact that it is all terribly ad hoc and that someone should do something to change that"*. Having a scientist as a vendor employee could give a totally different perspective to the whole sales and support process and may lead to a change of attitude towards the laboratory information system. Participant 21 added. *"The more that we (scientists) are involved, the more chance we have of making a system that does what we want—and that can bring about efficiencies like a paperless laboratory for instance"*.

4.7.5   Laboratory Information Systems Research in Private Pathology

The feelings of FG2 towards a lack of co-operation and synergy between the management, IT staff and scientists were the same as the researcher experienced with FG1—the public hospital laboratory. The participants' comments reflect the same lack of a cohesive approach to direction and planning in technical and IT services as seen in FG1. There is also a lack of awareness of such terms as "strategy, business–IT alignment and laboratory information system effectiveness". The question of research and education was raised by the researcher in the context that research and education in SISP would alleviate problems of lack of cohesion and foster worthwhile information system development. Participant 24 agreed that it would make a positive impact—*"research and education must be critically important to the development of medical science, and yet we have none in our course. And no-one researches laboratory information system that I know of"*. Lack of research and education in the area of medical informatics and SISP applied to the laboratory environment had led to stasis within the laboratory environment, as demonstrated by Participant 23– *"there is no information available to or passed on to we end-users and we have stagnated technically"*.

The participants of FG2 raised the issue of laboratory management in the context of a lack of formal courses for scientists who are to be promoted to middle management positions. As Participant 23 pointed out—*"being a good scientist does not make you a good manager. Management skills historically have been acquired by observation, not by education, and everyone does it differently"*. All participants strongly agreed that there should be formal management training for scientists who are being promoted to middle management and Participant 22 told the group that in his practice now there is an internal management course that is compulsory prior to promotion. He elaborated—*"we do some internal training now in budgets, cash flow and how to use spreadsheets to support this"*. Research and education in laboratory information system and technological IT advancements, and business processes such as SISP are nonexistent at this current point in time. The consensus (FG1 and FG2) is that there is a very considerable impediment to change in medical pathology information system in Australia.

4.7.6   Laboratory Information System Wish List—Private Pathology

The approach taken by the participants with respect to a laboratory information system wish list was to request small changes to their existing systems, such as alleviation of the problems associated with data entry by having the ability to digitise request slips. Participant 24 suggested—*"an automatic stock control system would be good—sort of a supply chain management system—so that we don't keep running out of reagents"*. More intelligence in the system was suggested by Participant 24 in the context of standardised, real time data and semi intelligent system to help interpret results—*"these things would save a lot of time for us"* he added.

It is interesting to note that responses of the participants of FG2, similar to those of FG1, did not include a consideration for a total change in the information system. For example, they did not consider a change to the adoption of a web-based information system. This similarity between the two groups is perhaps a reflection of a lack of knowledge of modern IT or the lack of the ability to laterally think to apply existing technologies to a different environment. The researcher initiated some discussion on web-based systems and what other technologies that are possible with a web-based system, for instance telemedicine, voice recognition software and voice over IP telephony. The participants reacted enthusiastically to the possibility of having these facilities and could appreciate their benefits. As Participant 24 noted—*"with the telemedicine, I could look at abnormal films from the country laboratories with the other scientists at the same time, in real time—instead of waiting two or three days for the films to get to me in Melbourne"*. The participants understood little of SISP, business–IT alignment and information system effectiveness measurement, which is understandable given the lack of education in these areas available to pathology staff. The impact of this lack of knowledge is evident from the discussion, as at no time during the focus group did any of the participants use terms such as "strategy, information system planning, information system effectiveness and business–IT alignment".

4.7.7 Summary

The key issues to emerge from the discussion of FG2 were similar to those main points that came from FG1. The main points from FG2, the private pathology laboratory were:

1. Co-operation between scientists, upper management and IT staff is virtually non-existent for the development of the laboratory information system;
2. Funding for laboratory development is based on minimal cost expenditure, and does not involve the laboratory information system;
3. There are no laboratory informatics or laboratory management courses available;
4. Conferences and the few papers that are published in medical science journals are concerned with middleware and not with the overt redevelopment of laboratory information system; and
5. The laboratory information system is not regarded in this case as an important part of the laboratory business by the upper management in private pathology.

4.8 Chapter Summary

The participants of FG1 and FG2 hold similar views on the proposals put to them in the focus group sessions. It is clear from the results of the analysis of both of the focus group data that the lack of financial support for laboratory information system development, along with a lack of laboratory information system capability, are the two main barriers to information system development in medical laboratories. It is interesting to note that, although the end results are similar between hospital and private pathology with respect to lack of spending, the mechanisms are quite different. The hospital laboratories are subject to internal (within the hospital) and external (government) politics and this determines the amount of financial support the laboratory receives. The private company wanting to maximise both profitability and shareholder returns, on the other hand, dictates spending in private pathology.

The FG1 and FG2 responses to the question of laboratory information system lack of capability suggest support for the conclusions that emerged from the survey. For example, the lack of capability of the laboratory information systems was reported by the participants to negatively impact on business outcomes because of an inability to integrate with modern communications technology, such as broadband e-mail and electronic ordering of pathology tests. End-users were not involved in the planning process with the result that workflow processes were compromised because of unsuitable or inadequate software development. The availability of finance for laboratory information system development was lacking in hospital pathology, as a result of the low priority with which the pathology is held within the hospital, and was lacking in private pathology because of the emphasis on maximising shareholder returns. Research and knowledge of formal business processes and current information systems technology compromised the pathology staff from both hospital and private laboratories in terms of creating development plans and to ascertain a future direction for the laboratory, should funding become available. There was no alignment between the business objectives of the practices and the direction of IT development, which negatively impacted on the laboratories abilities to service their respective referring practitioners.

The findings of this research have shown that the lack of laboratory information system capability results from an unwillingness of both the hospital and the private companies to invest in integration and monitoring of the information systems. In addition, there appear to be some political and policy issues affecting this situation. In the case of the public hospital pathology laboratory, both the attitude of the government towards health, and the attitude of the hospital CEO towards the pathology department reflect disinterest in laboratory development. The findings of FG1 showed that both of these forces were negative for the pathology department and that this compromised funding for the department. But an awareness of what is possible to have in a laboratory information system is also lacking in scientists in both the hospital and private pathology through lack of IT awareness of modern information systems technology and a closed view of current laboratory information systems. This was demonstrated by rejection of the idea of a web-based system and all that entails (for example—telemedicine, web-based voice recognition, paperless laboratory) in FG 1 and also by the participants of FG2 not including it on their IT wish list.

FG1 and FG2 participants had a closed view to the introduction of new IT. This was further demonstrated when all participants were asked about obtaining a new system—both groups as a whole started discussing the existing vendor systems and there was no mention of importing new technologies such as the web into their laboratory environments. The existing vendor systems are the same basic age as the technology that the hospital system currently uses. This outcome reflects a general lack of knowledge of research into new technologies within the pathology vertical in both hospital and private laboratories, and their possible application to medical laboratory IS. The current thrust of development in industry journals, the Clinical Biochemist Reviews for instance, is the implementation of auto-validation, a set of rules developed by pathology IT staff or IT vendor staff to validate test results automatically, to save the senior scientists and pathologists looking at results manually and validating these results.

Lack of cooperation between senior scientists in management positions (department heads) and IT staff has been shown by this research to play a significant role in ineffective laboratory information systems resulting in negative business outcomes for pathology, both private and hospital based. Examples of negative business outcomes for the hospital laboratory are a lack of ability to provide hospital doctors with electronic ordering of tests that has led to duplicate orders for tests due to slow turnaround time for results. There is also the loss of income from referring general practitioners because of the inability of the laboratory information system to accommodate broadband communications technology, precluding the laboratory from e-mailing results to the referring doctors. Examples of negative business outcomes for private pathology as a result of lack of capability of the laboratory information systems are the inability to create a paperless laboratory that would improve efficiencies and cost-effectiveness, and the lack of a web-based laboratory information system that would enable a better match between the laboratory information system and the private practice's global development.

The analysis of the focus group data has also highlighted another misalignment— that of scientist/management/IT. FG2 confirmed that this is more prevalent in the private practices surveyed where laboratory information system changes may be initiated by the IT staff alone, or with management—the scientists are rarely involved in discussion and planning of any changes. These changes are functional and not strategic and are frequently based on cost considerations. The researcher's experience that there is an IT staff attitude that scientists know nothing about IT has been confirmed in FG1 (p. 197). This attitude exists in spite of the fact that scientists are the main end-users and determine the workflow and what is required to support the work flow processes. The suggestion that IT staff thinks poorly of scientists' IT knowledge was also supported by the views expressed by the participants of FG2 (p. 207). This situation may result from a lack of knowledge and education on the part of all parties, and is further exacerbated by a lack of alignment between management, scientists and IT staff. To use the terminology seen in the SISP literature, there is a significant lack of business–IT alignment, compounded by non-existent end-user involvement in the planning process (Grover and Segars 2005; Chan et al. 2007; Rondeau et al. 2006; Jiang et al. 2002).

FG1 showed that because of the lack of funds, bought about by the low priority and lack of strategic capacity with which the hospital laboratory information system is held, there is an inability to change the laboratory information system to be more capable. Added to this, a lack of significant management data from the laboratory information system renders the hospital laboratory static. There are three major issues resulting from this:

1. Inability to provide a turnaround time for results commensurate with the acuteness of patients in ICU and CCU illnesses;
2. Inability to integrate developing technologies (communications) requested by referring practitioners which has led to a loss of work and income; and
3. Generation of excess work (over servicing) by doctors due to lack of availability of results in a timeframe similar to opposition practices—the doctors re-order the tests. This contradicts government efforts to cut health expenditure in the Australian context.

An unexpected consequence of the pressure of reduced staff numbers and the inadequate laboratory information system was raised by one participant—that of frustration and perhaps anger as the scientists have been aggressive when answering inquiries about result availability. The social aspects of this project are considerable and warrant further investigation, but do not apply to the research question of this current project. The researcher has mentioned this consequence to make the point that there are other manifestations of the lack of laboratory information system capability, the lack of finance and inadequate staffing levels. The scientists' attitudes can have a direct impact on the business, negative in this case:

- Too aggressive and rude behaviour may lead to loss of referrals and hence income; and
- May have an indirect negative financial impact through days lost with sick leave and the possible need for counselling (anger management).

The focus groups (FG1 and FG2) data suggest that the lack of laboratory information systems capability and effectiveness is having a negative impact on business outcomes for pathology in the Australian context. There is a demonstrable inability to undertake SISP. The key issues that emerged from the FGs affecting medical pathology information systems effectiveness are the lack of capability of the laboratory information systems, lack of business–IT alignment and poor end-user involvement and a low priority by the practice owners to finance developments in pathology information systems. There are three possible alternatives that laboratories could choose from to update their laboratory information system:

1. A commercial venture to build and implement the new system;
2. To form a consortium, as did the OpenLabs project. This could have additional benefits such as shared resources, central hosting of resources, better management of redundancy and disaster recovery and provision of a test environment (server compartment); and
3. The government could be involved through its Healthsmart project and in consultation with private and public pathology provide a standardised laboratory information system. This would be best configured as an application service provider (ASP) model where each laboratory could draw down modules to structure a unique system that best suited their own particular needs.

The data analysis of the two focus groups presented in this Chapter has supported the major findings of the quantitative data analysis (Chap. 5). The quantitative data analysis showed that laboratory information systems capability was the dominant mediator variable for SISP and that the survey participants viewed the laboratory information system as not capable of scalability and integration with modern technology. The focus group participants from both the hospital and private pathology sectors agreed that this lack of capability of the laboratory information system has had a negative impact on business outcomes for their respective laboratories. The participants' comments also confirmed that the laboratory information systems in both private and hospital laboratories were given little priority for development funding, due possibly to the supposition that the laboratory information systems are regarded as commodities.

The analysis of the survey data for the mediator variables—business–IT alignment and end-user involvement in planning—identified some recognition for these variables as a part of the process of laboratory information systems planning. The extent of the role played by business–IT alignment and end-user involvement was clarified by the participants of both focus groups who expressed a strong view that these two variables are important in the planning process. The participants went on to express strong disagreement that business–IT alignment and end-user involvement in planning took place in either hospital or private laboratories and that this negatively impacts the effectiveness of the laboratory information systems.

The participants of FG1 and FG2 acknowledged that there is no funding for the strategic development of laboratory information systems in their respective laboratories, as was shown in the quantitative analysis results. The participants' suggestion for this observation was that funding is functional and not strategic. This would explain the marked change in the multiple regression beta weights between the first and second regressions that were obtained.

The focus groups discussed in this Chapter have provided rich data to complement the findings of the survey analysis presented in Chap. 5. There are, however, some findings that are yet to be fully explained—in particular the concept of functional and not strategic funding and what underlies this concept, and the possibility and extent to which the laboratory information system is regarded as a commodity. These incomplete findings form the basis for the more specialised discussion and interpretation that follows in Chap. 6 where another focus group was established to deepen the researcher's understanding of these issues.

Chapter 5
Focus Group 3: The Experts

5.1 Introduction

This chapter reports an analysis of a third focus group of academicians and practitioners experienced in Strategic Information Systems Planning (SISP) who discussed the ramifications of the outcomes of the focus groups in the two practitioner sites reported in Chap. 4.

The expected linear multiple regression results supported the original contentions of this study that financial considerations (cost–benefit analysis—Saarinen 1996; Lincoln 1986; Mayer 1998), end-user involvement in planning (Rondeau et al. 2006; Hackney and Kawalek 1999) and business–IT alignment (Chan and Reich 2007; Delone and McLean 1992, 2003; Segars and Grover 2005) are the major issues affecting the outcome of SISP. The unexpected findings were a marked decrease in beta weights from the first regression (independent variables of financial considerations, business–IT alignment and end-user involvement against the mediator variables) to the second regression (mediator variables against the dependent variable SISP). The beta score for pathology information systems capability was consistently the highest beta value, and therefore, it can be argued, has the greatest influence on the dependent variable SISP. The ability for pathology laboratories to undertake SISP, it was argued in Chaps. 2 and 3, is a pre-requisite for information systems effectiveness measurement and hence the measurement of business outcomes.

The participants of FG1 and FG2 had also raised the possibility that the changes observed in the quantitative data analysis for financial considerations may be because spending is functional; the strategic ramifications of this view will be explored in this chapter with particular reference to impact of decisions about functional spending on SISP and business outcomes for the pathology industry. The participants in both FG1 and FG2 also observed that the pathology information systems are viewed as a commodity in both hospital and private pathology, but could not fully explain why. They did, however, acknowledge that the current management perspectives towards the pathology laboratories have a negative impact on strategic planning and business outcomes. Although the extent to which end-users are involved in planning and the degree of business–IT alignment was not fully explained by the data obtained from

M. Belkin et al., *Strategic ICT Planning in Pathology,*
Healthcare Delivery in the Information Age,
DOI 10.1007/978-1-4614-4478-7_5, © Springer Science+Business Media, LLC 2013

Table 5.1 Academic focus group participant details

Participant	Description and qualifications
Participant 31	Professor of management information systems, Head of school, Dean of research and innovation
Participant 32	Post doctoral strategy consultant
Participant 33	Post doctoral—senior lecturer alignment
Participant 34	Post doctoral—researcher SISP and statistical methods
Participant 35	Post doctoral—thesis on SISP in Australia
Participant 36	Doctoral candidate—researching alignment

FG1 and FG2, the participants supported the contention that these were essential for effective planning to occur.

A focus group of SISP experts was seen as an efficient way to stimulate discussion on the quantitative data analysis and FG1 and FG2 findings to try and elicit an explanation for these anomalies and assess their impact on understanding an answer to study the main issue *"How does the effectiveness of laboratory information systems impact on business outcomes in medical pathology in Australia?"*

5.2 Focus Group of Experts

The participants invited to attend the focus group were six in number (seven including the researcher). Six of the participants are academics (one professor and five post doctoral) within a research school at RMIT University, Australia, and the seventh is a doctorally qualified consultant in the health vertical for a multinational consulting firm (Table 5.1). All members of the panel have practical experience with SISP applications in industries. Only two have actual experience in the health vertical.

As a prelude to the commencement of discussion on the anomalies seen in the multiple regressions, the researcher gave the experts participating in FG3 an overview of pathology laboratories, in both the business and IT contexts. As a result of this overview, a discussion developed which focused on a set of key issues and explanations that emerged which the panel considered were significant in the context of this research.

The key issues arising from the study process as a result of the survey and the two focus groups of pathology practitioners are that:

- There is a lack of funding for pathology laboratory development, including laboratory information systems development.
- There is a lack of end-user involvement in the planning process in pathology laboratories.
- There is a lack of business–IT alignment in the planning process in pathology laboratories.
- Laboratory information system capability is the major influencing mediator variable on SISP in pathology.

- Research and education into pathology laboratory management and information systems does not occur.
- There is no awareness of the principles of SISP in the pathology industry.

Each of these issues was put to the panel of experts and the results of their analysis are discussed in detail in the following section.

5.3 Strategic Impact, Alignment and Commoditisation

The researcher explained to the participants of FG3 that this study is interested in determining the role that the recognised contributors to successful strategic planning (business–IT alignment, end-user involvement and financial considerations) play in pathology. Successful SISP is seen as a cohesive approach to strategic planning and each component plays a pivotal role without which SISP is compromised. He acknowledged that analysis of FG1 and FG2 has shown some of the components to be lacking, notably business–IT alignment and end-user involvement, but the full understanding of the research findings and their impact on SISP needed to be elicited by the SISP experts of FG3.

The researcher initiated discussion in FG3 with the statement and question—*"we found a high beta value for laboratory information systems capability against SISP compared to business–IT alignment and end-user involvement that is in the classical literature—what are your comments and feedback on that—what do you think that might mean?"* To inform the participants of FG3 of the views held by the members of the two previous FGs with respect to an assessment of the strategic value of the pathology information system, the researcher explained—*"Focus Group 1 (FG1) showed that there is apparently no strategy in pathology test request and no priority given to strategic development of pathology in hospital funding, yet the pathology test results in many cases (intensive care, cardiac unit and emergency) are required quickly and accurately for treatment and diagnosis of desperately ill patients"* (Chap. 4). Participant 31 reiterated the scientists' view—*"scientists don't care about strategy. They are not involved in any planning; there is no end-user involvement so over the years they have lost interest. The hospital doctors don't understand about SISP—the words are not known to them and neither are the principles. There is a misalignment of the knowledge domains".*

The participants then sought an explanation for this observation, Participant 31 commenting that—*"the survey involved educated people, many with PhDs— pathologists and medical scientists, yet you got an incredibly low r^2 value for research and education for SISP—it is almost as though none of that matters at all".* Participant 33 asked the question—*"is the low beta value due to lack of research and education in the field of pathology laboratory information systems—could that have a negative impact on strategy for pathology"?*

The participants acknowledged that there is little or no research or education in pathology information systems in Australia. There is an undergraduate course in pathology informatics and laboratory management available at the researcher's university and for which the researcher teaches. The researcher explained that the course content does not contain any material on SISP, information systems effectiveness measurement or pathology information systems development, and went on to add that—*"there is no material on strategy, strategic planning or strategic development and effectiveness measurement of pathology information systems"*. It was proposed by Participant 31 that scientists and medical people do not understand SISP and that a lack of research and education relevant to SISP has a negative impact on the performance and business outcomes of laboratories in both hospital and private pathology. Participant 31 added, for the hospital laboratory —*"the lack of strategy, planning and of pathology information system development is such that the pathology information systems cannot perform basic function such as electronic ordering of tests in the wards. Data entry is so slow that the laboratory can have a test result before the patient details are entered in the computer—the ward has to wait for the results. There is no strategic planning and the information system is not effective"*.

The participants noted in their discussion that lack of strategic planning is an example of one of the problems that pathology laboratories in general face. The FG3 participants acknowledged that lack of research and education and lack of end-user involvement in planning contribute to this, but still does not give a full explanation for the attitude held by scientists, hospital management and doctors alike that the pathology information systems have no strategic value. This research has shown that there is no provision of finance for strategic development of the pathology information systems. The participants in FG3 agreed that this is due to the fact that the pathology information system is regarded as a commodity in both the hospital and the private pathology environments and as such is seen to have no strategic value. Participant 34 expressed this succinctly—*"pathology information systems have been commoditised to such a degree that they just are looking at outcomes not strategies—that's all. For laboratories to spend an unknown amount for an unknown outcome is a big risk when they now have something dependable and predictable—establishing a connection between business outcomes and pathology information systems is the real trick, and in fact what your research is probably doing is establishing that this connection does not exist"*.

Participant 33 made the further observation that management of both hospital and private pathology appears to prioritise the accounts/financial functions and any perceived management functions of the pathology information systems because these areas are seen as areas of income production. Participant 34 noted that—*"the accounts department is seen to produce cold hard cash—spending in the laboratory would produce small intangible benefits only, and these would be very difficult to measure"*. Participant 33 added—*"hospital funding in Australia is based on case mix principles—that is patients in beds. The priority of hospital management is turnover of patients—there is no metric for better patient outcomes. There is no tie back to the actual business with pathology—there is no metric to say that if the hospital had a good pathology service that it would result in better patient outcomes"*.

Following intense discussion about the issues raised above, the participants came to a conclusion that the hospital management apparently does not make the connection because of the commoditisation[1] of the pathology information systems and services. Commoditisation in this context relates to the definition given below, derived from a member of FG3. The nature of this commoditisation can be illustrated by a comment from Participant 31 who noted that—*"pathology is fundamental to the investigation of disease—but it is not seen as strategic in any way, shape or form, but it is fundamental to the process"*. Participant 33 further added—*"It would be a subtle point to justify spending on the laboratory information systems in hospitals because of this view"*.

The participants in FG3 noted that there is an enigma concerning the attitude with which pathology is held. Participant 32 explained—*"there is no recognition of the possibility that, with improved technology and information system effectiveness at some cost and effective planning, the pathology services could be delivered in a more timely and efficient manner"*. This, the participants noted, surely must contribute to better patient care and perhaps faster recovery and earlier discharge—hence enhancing the probability of a higher turn-around of patients and the attraction of more funds under the case mix funding process. The proposition put forward by the participants that the hospital pathology information systems is widely regarded as a commodity and as such has no strategic value would then explain why the pathology information systems have seemingly no priority when it comes to the provision of funds by hospital management for its development. This view was described by Participant 33—*"This situation is compounded in no small way by the attitude that the pathology information systems is a commodity—in the mind of management it is not seen to exist"*.

The participants' proposition that the pathology information system is a commodity would also contribute to understanding why there is no active development of the pathology information systems in private practice pathology laboratories. Funding is fundamental, but not strategic, for the diagnosis of disease. This was stated bluntly by Participant 34—*"the laboratories are pushed out as far as possible from high priority—they are a commodity"*. The researcher expanded on one element affecting management's apparent attitude towards pathology by mentioning the coning rules[2] as applied by Medicare (Australia's public healthcare system)—*"under the coning rules, private pathology suffers most. They are only paid for the three most expensive blood tests under these rules and if doctors order more than three tests, they don't get paid for them"*. The participants in FG3 then agreed that these coning rules contribute to an apparent explanation for the observed managerial attitudes within the health vertical and contribute to the problems of lack of strategic development and capability that beset pathology laboratory information systems. The observed anomalies

---

[1] Commoditisation may be defined as "The process whereby product selection becomes more dependent on price than differentiating features, benefits and value added services." (sensacom.com/web_glossary.html)

[2] Coning rules are part of the Federal government Health policy relating to pathology testing in Australia. The coning rules apply to general practitioners ordering blood tests on non hospitalised patients, and allow for payment of the three most expensive tests ordered to the pathology practice. Test numbers in excess of three tests are not paid under the coning rules.

in the quantitative data analysis, that is, the dramatic change in beta weights of the financial considerations variables and the consistently higher score for laboratory expandability and adaptability over business–IT alignment, however, are in the opinions of the FG3 participants, still not fully accounted for, but some conclusions could be supported.

As a result of the pathology information systems being viewed as a commodity, the following observations have support in the research data:

- The pathology information system does not have any strategic value.
- The pathology information system does not attract developmental spending.
- The scientists have lost interest in pathology information systems and laboratory development in general.
- There is no encouragement or incentive to undertake research and education on pathology information system involvement in SISP/strategic development of laboratory.

A detailed discussion on the attitudes to spending in both hospital and private pathology follows.

5.4   Functional Versus Strategic Spending

The researcher reported to the FG3 participants that the conclusion made from the multiple regression results, combined with his laboratory experience in a senior departmental management role; suggests that there is no financial expenditure on pathology information systems expansion in a strategic sense in Australia. The researcher asked the participants to consider the data analysis pertaining to private pathology (Chap. 5) that showed for the initial multiple regression of the three independent variables "financial data valuable", "information format", and "information underlies change" against the mediator variable "financial information", the independent variable "information underlies change" had the highest beta score; in fact, it had the only significant score. This suggests, argued the researcher in FG3, that the financial information in private pathology underlies change. However, when the mediator variable, "financial information" was regressed against the SISP dependent variable, the beta score changed dramatically and became insignificant. This is a highly significant and unexpected finding when compared to other industry verticals studied in the research literature (Lincoln 1986; Sugumaran and Arogyaswamy 2004; Irani and Love 2001). This, the researcher argued to the FG3 experts, suggests that unique to the pathology industry, the financial considerations are internal, that is, the financial considerations underlie change, but the change is functional, not strategic. The discussion on this proposition amongst the participants of FG3 was initiated when the researcher asked the group—*"given what is coming out in the discussion here and that the analysis findings are starting to be explained—do you think that the laboratory information system can be viewed by private pathology as a component of SISP?"*

Participant 31 began the discussion noting that—*"when you talk about SISP it just doesn't connect in a medical environment because it is not seen as strategy—it is just seen as a commodity. The pathology information system has no priority as it is not seen as a strategic tool—it is seen as a commodity"*. Expenditure in private pathology laboratories, the participants concluded, is therefore functional spending, not strategic spending. The underlying consideration to spending in private pathology is cost cutting, not strategic development. Participant 33 added another perspective on the strategic ability of laboratories in the context of business–IT alignment by commenting that—*"the range of the cognitive gap between PC and mainframe is twenty five years of technology. IT should be business driven with IT going along for the ride—it should be their desire to become more up to date and have access to opportunities they would otherwise not have—if IT is driving this, it is almost doomed to failure. You would think that business and IT would want to be on the same page"*.

The researcher then raised another issue relating to strategic development in private pathology; that being the drive for international expansion by two of the three major private pathology practices in Australia. Participant 32 commented—*"One would think there would be pressure brought to bear on these laboratories because of their overseas expansion—the introduction of such capabilities as a web based pathology information systems with intranets and internets for improved and real-time communication, telemedicine for real-time review of cases from anywhere in the world and web based voice recognition software to eliminate transcription should provide a strategic advantage"*. Participant 35 commented—*"One would think that the laboratory management would find this not only attractive, but essential for growth"*.

The discussion by the SISP experts in FG3 relating to functional versus strategic spending has highlighted that both hospital and private pathology do not perceptibly undertake strategic spending. This was also supported by the analysis of the survey and demonstrated in that analysis by the marked decrease in beta weights for financial information between the first and second regressions. The discussion in FG1, FG2 and FG3 has also contributed to the understanding of why strategic spending does not occur in either hospital or private pathology in terms of what influences spending in each environment. In the hospital environment, the management of the hospital and the incumbent political party's view on health spending determines spending. Private pathology spending is concerned with cost cutting and maximising shareholder returns. Underlying both these scenarios is the fact that the pathology information systems in both hospital and private pathology are regarded as a commodity. The participants of FG3 acknowledge that the combination of functional spending and the pathology information systems being viewed as a commodity in this way has a significant negative impact on pathology's ability to undertake SISP, and this is demonstrated practically in the example relating to international expansion given above.

Again not all issues raised from the survey research or all of the outcomes from FG1 and FG2 had been dealt with by FG3 up to this point. The degree of pathology information systems capability that is present in current pathology information systems needed to be explored, especially since this variable was shown by the regressions to have the most influence on SISP in pathology, and the discussion of what emerged in FG3 is reported in the following section.

5.5 Information System Functionality Versus Information System Capability

The participants acknowledged that what is under investigation in this study is the capability of the pathology information system, not its functionality, and its impact on SISP. They further noted that there is a difference between capability and functionality and to make this distinction has some ramifications, not only for the pathology industry, but also for some established business–IT models. One of the FG3 experts referred to one such model that of Henderson and Venkatraman (1993) which the study had already prepared to test as it was a key part of the initial research, reported in Chap. 2.

After distributing a diagram of the Henderson and Venkatraman strategic alignment model (1993), the researcher asked the group to explore the possible interpretation of the pathology information systems capability in the context of the strategic alignment model (SAM) to obtain a total understanding of its impact on SISP and to help align the findings of this study with the established literature. The researcher asked—*"if one considers the Henderson and Venkatraman strategic alignment model in light of my second multiple regression findings—the IT strategy involves technical scope, IT governance, system competencies, IT architecture, processes and skills—these could be classified as functional components of an IT system. Does the result of the multiple regression, that is, the dominance of pathology information systems capability suggest another component of their model hitherto unconsidered—information systems capability?"* (Fig. 5.1)

The researcher described the model, saying—*"In the SAM, all four sections interact in the model to produce a cohesive, multi-dimensional relationship with good strategic fit. Each section and sub-section is dependent on the other components of the model for a complete business-IT relationship and successful and on-going alignment"*. Participant 34 commented—*"in the context of the findings in your research, one of the sub-sections, that of systemic competencies, which embraces what competencies of IT strategy can contribute positively to the creation of new business strategies, or better support existing strategies, has been shown to be lacking. This is due to a view held by the health vertical in general that the pathology information system is a commodity, is not a strategic tool and therefore does not warrant allocation of funds for development and enhancement. In this context the SAM fails in pathology"*.

The participants then discussed the concept that a system may be functional, but not capable, and the ramifications for SISP and business outcomes in pathology. An example was given by the researcher—*"The current pathology information systems, as used in private and hospital laboratories alike, has the functionality to accept*

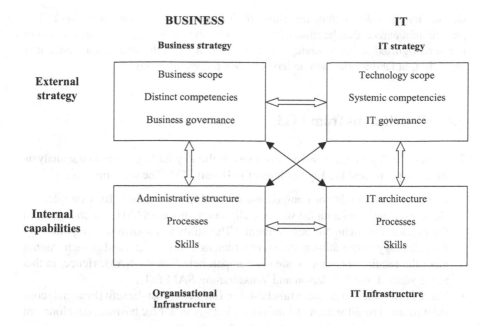

Fig. 5.1 Henderson and Venkatraman strategic alignment model (adapted from Henderson and Venkatraman 1993)

patient demographic information to identify patient results through unique identifiers, and place the results in the patient files for reporting. The current pathology information systems can provide laboratory and management staff with data such as patient numbers for individual doctors, test numbers and limited financial data. These examples of pathology information systems functionality have not changed or developed significantly since the pathology information systems were written". Participant 36 added—*"Pathology information system capability, for example, could involve modern technologies such as telemedicine, wireless communications technology, voice recognition software, local area networks for dissemination of analyser graphics and the realisation of a paperless laboratory to mention but a few. This would then allow for strategic expansion that is just not possible now".*

Following lengthy discussion, the participants in FG3 then agreed to one proposal that it is this lack of capability over the last 25 years or so since information systems were introduced to pathology laboratories, which has led to the attitude now commonly held by scientists and management alike—that the pathology information system is a commodity. As such the pathology information system has no strategic value and cannot be regarded as a component of SISP. Participant 32 asked—*"do people, because the pathology information system is inflexible and not able to change, and because they are not involved in planning, draw the line then and say we can't do anything and throw their hands in the air and not bother?"* The participants agreed that because of this attitude, the pathology information system is not recognised as being strategic now nor will it be in the future, and hence it is unlikely that laboratories will undertake any strategic planning.

5.6 Conclusions from FG3

The aim of FG3 was to investigate and explore the key findings of both the analysis of the survey data and the key findings of FG1 and FG2. The outcomes are:

*   The relevance/weight for components of established models, for example, the Henderson and Venkatraman strategic alignment model (SAM) may change from the expected in niche business verticals. The study has shown that in pathology the pathology information system is regarded as a commodity, and as such, cannot meet the requirements for "systemic competencies" of the SAM. Hence, in this niche vertical, the Henderson and Venkatraman SAM fails.
*   There is a distinction between functional and strategic cost–benefit (financial) considerations. The allocation of funds in pathology is not for business development or expansion and hence cannot be viewed as strategic.
*   There is a distinction between information system functionality and capability. The current lack of capability of the pathology laboratory information systems to integrate with modern technology and to provide flexibility and scalability to enhance the strategic development of the business is confirmed by this study.
*   The pathology information system is widely regarded in both hospital and private pathology as a commodity, and as such has no strategic value or competency. This prevents SISP, information system effectiveness and the strategic development of medical pathology.
*   The pathology information system capability was found to be the overriding factor in laboratory strategic development. This study has shown a variance from the expected insignificance of the recognised contributors to successful SISP (financial considerations, end-user involvement and business-IT alignment) as explained above and in the context of the peculiarities of the niche vertical of medical pathology. Therefore the degree of capability of the pathology information systems directly impacts with business outcomes in medical pathology. This study has shown that impact to be negative.
*   SISP cannot take place in pathology laboratories. This study shows that there is no means by which pathology laboratories are able to do so. There are no research and education activities to keep staff abreast of developing technology and strategies for development; a lack of information system capability overrides the possibility of successful business–IT alignment; there is no strategic spending; end users are not involved in any planning or development exercises.

Chapter 6
Discussion and Conclusion

6.1 Overview

The aim of this research was to establish whether the effectiveness of pathology information systems impacts on business outcomes in pathology practice in Australia. This study is breaking new ground, as there is no evidence in the literature that a study of this kind has been done before in the pathology industry. In this chapter, there is also discussion of issues that arise from the research findings, and their implications for both practitioners and academics are highlighted. These implications are particularly important for practitioners as the study offers the potential for the development of diagnostic tools that could provide a more standardised approach to strategic planning of information systems and information systems effectiveness measurement models.

This research has evolved the strategic information systems planning/information systems (SISP/IS) effectiveness composite model as a contribution to the development of diagnostic tools for SISP and information systems effectiveness measurement. This model combines the principles of SISP as a pre-cursor to the assessment of information systems effectiveness measurement on the basis that a project needs to undertake a properly structured SISP before the project effectiveness can be assessed. The SISP/IS effectiveness composite model then uses the achievement of a carefully researched and established business goal as the measure of information systems effectiveness. A diagrammatic representation of the SISP/IS effectiveness model is seen in Fig. 6.1.

The commitment to both a wide area of investigation, to provide a holistic perspective on the effectiveness of information systems in pathology and their impact on strategic planning of information systems and business outcomes, and a micro-analysis, to investigate the content of relations between variables, yields a number of research limitations. These limitations are discussed in this chapter. The research process revealed some issues that could not be tested within this study. These issues are detailed as limitations and together with the findings of the research are put as suggestions for future research at the end of the chapter.

M. Belkin et al., *Strategic ICT Planning in Pathology,*
Healthcare Delivery in the Information Age,
DOI 10.1007/978-1-4614-4478-7_6, © Springer Science+Business Media, LLC 2013

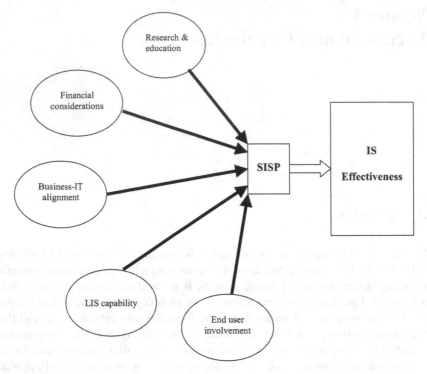

Fig. 6.1 SISP/IS effectiveness composite model

6.1.1 The Process

A unifying "process map" shows the navigation of this study, and this chapter draws on all four elements in that process map—the literature review, a survey, two industry focus groups and a focus group of experts—to derive a set of findings and conclusions. The research developed out of the researcher's own experience working in medical science. There was an obvious problem with pathology laboratories and information systems used in them. The researcher had tried to develop an alternative information system but this too had failed to attract any attention. The research began by investigating the existing literature and uncovering almost no research on pathology information systems. A subsequent investigation of the literature on information systems development and planning resulted in a review of current knowledge and research about strategic planning and SISP. This was then used to form a theoretical grounding for the research and existing models were adapted as a framework to underpin the research process. In addition, the very small amount of research in this area was then used to extend that model. Key principles of SISP—business–IT alignment, end-user involvement in planning and financial consideration in planning—were wedded with two other concepts to frame the research.

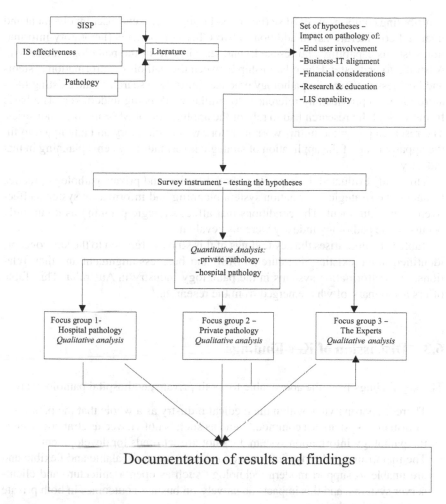

Fig. 6.2 The research process

Two periods of research activity—a survey, followed by three focus groups—were used to build enough data to develop an answer for the research question "How does the effectiveness of laboratory information systems impact on business outcomes in medical pathology practice"? The process map is illustrated in Fig. 6.2.

The conclusions derived from the analysis of the data collected are described in the next section.

6.2 Key Findings

The aim of the study was to determine the level of strategic information systems planning and by what means information systems effectiveness is measured in private and public hospital pathology practices in Australia. The research utilised existing contributing components of SISP (business–IT alignment, end-user involvement and financial considerations) in addition to two other components (laboratory information systems capability and research) and tested them in the pathology industry in Australia to understand the relationship between the pathology information systems and business outcomes in pathology practice. Initially, a search of the existing literature failed to provide any references to similar work being undertaken. The basic framework of the research had to rely of the application of SISP in other industries. The research presented in this work therefore was exploratory and attempted to fill the apparent gap of the application of strategic information systems planning in that industry.

This study evaluated the capacity of both hospital and private pathology practice to undertake strategic information system planning and information systems effectiveness measurement. The conditions that affect strategic planning as it currently occurs in the pathology industry were also evaluated.

Table 6.1 summarises the key findings of this study in relation to the key concepts identified in the existing literature on SISP and business alignment and their relationship to information systems in the pathology industry in Australia. This Table offers a summary of what emerged from the research.

6.3   Discussion of Key Findings

The key findings from the above table for both private and hospital pathology are:

- There is a strong view within the medical industry as a whole that the pathology information system is a commodity and as such is not viewed as strategic. Hence the pathology information system does not attract funds for development.
- The mainframe pathology information systems are not scalable and flexible and are unable to support modern technology such as open architecture and client-server systems, and this impacts negatively on business outcomes in both private and hospital pathology.
- The pathology information systems were found to be functional and not strategic which compounded their lack of scalability and flexibility.
- There is no objective means of measuring and evaluating information systems planning effectiveness used by the private or hospital pathology.
- Spending on investment in pathology in both private and hospital pathology is functional and not strategic.
- Business–IT alignment and end-user involvement in strategic planning are not evident in either private or hospital pathology.
- The presence of a monopoly in private pathology practice negatively influences information systems development in both private and hospital pathology.
- Middle management in both private and hospital pathology practice is not IT aware, and the IT staff in both private and hospital pathology are not familiar with the business and strategic goals of the firm.

Table 6.1 A summary of the comparable findings in the literature review and data analysis

Key concepts	Research literature source	Existing research findings	Pathology IS research findings and comments (related to this present study)
Business–IT alignment	Henderson & Venkatraman (1993); Grover & Segars (2005); Burn & Szeto (2000); Chan et al. (1997); King (1998); Chen & Reich (2007)	Business–IT alignment is inherently of value and contributes to the organisation's success; Success comes from linking the IT plan to the business plan and this ensures congruence between business strategy and IT strategy; Organisations that align business strategy and IT strategy outperform those that do not align	Business–IT alignment was not evident in this study in the pathology industry; This study found that there was little alignment with respect to business objectives between scientists, management and the demands on IT in pathology laboratories; This research found little evidence of business–IT alignment in either private or hospital pathology
Business–IT alignment and competitive advantage	Wang & Tai (2003); Rondeau (2006)	Business–IT alignment creates competitive advantage for the firm; Alignment requires continuous assessment by the firm to keep competitive advantage	There was poor awareness by stakeholders of the link between alignment and competitive advantage in pathology found by this study; This research found no evidence of Business–IT alignment in pathology
IT/IS in pathology	Wells et al. (1996); Bender and McNair (1996); Boran et al. (1996); Anandarajan & Arinze (1998)	A lack of IS development has the pathology industry lagging behind other knowledge-based verticals; The OpenLabs project is an example of the application of SISP principles in pathology—a planning exercise using all the principles of SISP to achieve an established business goal; Open architecture systems and Client server systems have been shown to increase flexibility and scalability into pathology IS resulting in enhanced business planning capability such as matching the organisation's information processing needs and interoperability	This research confirms that pathology IS development is lagging behind other knowledge-based verticals; This research showed that none of the principles of SISP were evident in private or hospital pathology practice; This research showed that the pathology IS in use in the examples sampled in this study are unable to support modern technology such as open architecture and client server systems, and that the mainframe systems in use are not scalable and flexible
Alignment mechanism and measurement	Kearns & Lederer (2000); Chan et al. (1997)	Successful planning is enhanced by organisational leaders knowledge of IT; IT leaders should understand corporate strategy to ensure planning success	This research found that leaders in pathology have a poor knowledge of IT and/or strategy, and do not communicate with other stakeholders or co-plan with the end users; This research found that IT leaders in the pathology industry in Australia have a poor understanding of strategy

Table 6.1 (continued)

Key concepts	Research literature source	Existing research findings	Pathology IS research findings and comments (related to this present study)
SISP	Grover & Segars (2005); Earl (1993); Sullivan (1985); Sabherwal & King (1995); Boynton & Zmud (1987); Zmud et al. (1986); Lederer & Sethi (1998)	The application of SISP principles to planning gives competitive advantage by enabling existing business strategies, improving customer satisfaction, enabling superior capabilities, providing advantage at lower cost and creating new business strategies	The principles that underlie SISP are not evident in either the hospital or private pathology laboratories in this study
		SISP involves a rational and structured approach that was found to be more effective and adaptable than highly structured approaches in the planning process	This study has shown that there is no structured approach to planning in private or hospital pathology
End-user involvement in planning	Sabherwal & King (1995); Grover & Segars (2005); Jaing et al. (2002); Hackney et al. (1999)	End-user involvement helps to overcome business–IT misalignment by improving internal communication, enabling existing business strategies, providing better understanding of IT/IS potential and enhancing the quality of decision support	This study found that end users are not involved in planning—and that this compromises IS development, and leads to poor understanding of IS potential, poor decision making, compromised service quality and negatively impacts on business outcomes
		Empowerment of end users and a feeling of ownership helps the planning process and gives positive impression of IS that enhances its use	The study showed through lack of end-user involvement there was a lack of a feeling of ownership by the participants and this established a negative attitude towards the pathology IS and a lack of interest in its use
SISP models	Nolan (1979); Porter & Miller (1985); Applegate et al. (1996); Greiner (1972); Wang & Tai (2003); Magal et al. (1998)	Nolan's growth model—Six stages of growth—initiation, contagion, control, integration, data administration, maturity. This model represents a growth and learning model for organisations implementing IS to obtain success	The existing models, i.e. Henderson and Venkatraman SAM, Delone and McLean success model, Wang and Tai organisational context model, Petter et al. and Porter and Miller life cycle concept model were found not to have little applicability in the private or hospital pathology sites studied
		Life cycle concept model—This model illustrates how businesses develop and adapt through pressure on the business	This study found that the life cycle concept model was not evident in practice in either the private or hospital pathology laboratories studied

Table 6.1 (continued)

Key concepts	Research literature source	Existing research findings	Pathology IS research findings and comments (related to this present study)
		Learning from crisis model—a model that demonstrates how businesses undertake learning and adapting through business crisis survival	This research found no evidence of the existence of crisis model learning in either the private or hospital pathology laboratories studied
		Information centres evolving by learning and adapting from clients ultimately become a corporate resource	There was no evidence for the existence of learning centres in private or hospital pathology in this research
		Evolution of growth through slack' and "control"—to achieve technology assimilation and to learn how to use new technologies more effectively	This research found that there were no methods of technology assimilation used in either private or hospital pathology laboratories studied
		Impacts of organisational contexts, content and process dimensions and planning system's capability are pivotal to successful IS planning	There was no evidence of the consideration of organisational contexts, process dimensions and planning system capabilities in either of the planning process in private or hospital pathology laboratories studied
IS evaluation	Irani & Love (2001); Symons (1991); Klecun & Cornford (2005); Grover et al. (1998); Smithson & Hirschheim (1998); Bannister & Remenyi (2000); Walsham (1993); Renkema & Berghout (1997); Forbes et al. (1999); Irani & Love (2002); Seymour (1991)	The difficulties of evaluation of IT/IS benefits were found to be excessive cost, extensive time frame and existing methods that are ineffective in the evaluation of IS projects/systems	This study found that IS evaluation of pathology information systems is tenuous and is based on the functional requirements of the laboratory and not related to any strategic capability of the information systems. The research also found that scientists evaluated the development of a new technologically capable pathology IS as too expensive
		The conditions for evaluation need to be defined to consider personal agendas and bias, that is, there needs to be an evaluation context established for meaningful evaluation	This research found that there were management personal agendas and internal politics operating in public hospitals and this contributed to the pathology IS being evaluated as having little priority for planning and development. Pathology IS were evaluated poorly in the hospital environment compared to other organisational structures

Table 6.1 (continued)

Key concepts	Research literature source	Existing research findings	Pathology IS research findings and comments (related to this present study)
IS evaluation (continued)		IS evaluation in health vertical is difficult because of complexity of industry, number of stakeholders and different organisational structures within related components of the industry	Consideration for investor stakeholders was given precedence in private pathology IS evaluation rather than investment in what they viewed as risky new ISThe research found that there was a stratification of personal evaluation of the pathology IS by different stakeholders for differing personal and/or political reasons
		The emphasis on organisational change has introduced political, cultural and organisational aspects in the evaluation process that may influence the evaluative outcome to be incomplete, biased or superficial	This research found no evidence of IS evaluation tools or process in pathology
		There is difficulty in assessing measuring tools for evaluation—traditionally technical aspects of a system have been evaluated but more recently organisational change aspects are being considered as at least equally important	This research has identified a void between pathology and other business verticals in terms of the knowledge and application of organisational elements of IS and their consideration in the evaluation process
		The literature highlights contradictions of outcomes with respect to the relationship between IT/IS investments and organisational productivity, and how this is measured	This research demonstrated some contradictions in the evaluation of the pathology IS in that productivity was measured as applicable to one functional component of the pathology IS and did not relate to the evaluation to overall organisational productivity

Table 6.1 (continued)

Key concepts	Research literature source	Existing research findings	Pathology IS research findings and comments (related to this present study)
IS effectiveness measurement	Grover & Segars (2005); Raghunathan & Raghunathan (1988); Premkumar & King (1992); Lederer & Sethi (1998); Youthas & Young (1998); Gation (1994); Grover et al. (1998); Saarinen (1996); Petter et al. (2008); Lincloln (1986); Parasuraman (1985); Pitt et al. (2001); Delone & McLean (1992); Petter et al. (2008); Petter et al. (2008); Molla & Licker (2001); Delone & McLean (2004)	Measurement of IS effectiveness methods commonly involves IS use, user information satisfaction (UIS), and decision support capability	There was no objective means of assessing pathology IS effectiveness identified in this study in either private or hospital pathology
		There is controversy relating to UIS as a measure of IS effectiveness as it is debated whether UIS is a true indicator of IS effectiveness	The controversy surrounding the use of UIS as a measure of IS effectiveness was encountered in this research in the context of recognition by participants that the pathology IS provided UIS for some functional data provision. There was, however, overall agreement by participants that the same data provision was not strategic and could not be used to assess IS effectiveness strategically
		Inefficient IS effectiveness measurement is due to the shortcomings of UIS as measure of IS effectiveness—UIS is a behavioural/attitude phenomena and has little relationship with primary business goals	This research revealed evidence that UIS is a personal view of the effectiveness of the pathology IS and as such did not relate to the business goals of the firms in this study
		SESAME—represents another method of IS effectiveness measurement and is based on cost-benefit analysis. It has contributed to a more rational approach to IS effectiveness measurement by using a standardised methodology	Functional decisions based on cost-benefit analysis and other financial considerations were found to occur in pathology IS development but were found not to apply to strategic development of pathology IS and its effectiveness assessment in either public or private laboratories in this research
		SERVQUAL—represents another means of standardised assessment of IS effectiveness and measures IT department service quality as opposed to assessing applications	This study identified a lack of an objective and formal method of assessing service quality in pathology
		The six dimension success model—system quality, information quality, service quality use, user satisfaction and net benefits are a basis for IS effectiveness measurement	This research found that the use of models for the assessment of IS effectiveness did not occur in pathology and that participants in the study were unaware of their existence
		The Delone and McLean success model has been expanded to include the impact of service quality, knowledge management and e-commerce in response to the changing components and means of doing business	Knowledge management methods were found not to exist in pathology. The lack of pathology IS capability was found to exclude pathology from developing an e-commerce component to its business model(s)

Table 6.1 (continued)

Key concepts	Research literature source	Existing research findings	Pathology IS research findings and comments (related to this present study)
Composite planning models	Singh (1993); Zhu & Kraemer (2005)	Most planning models incorporate strategic, tactical and operational levels, and have provision for an external feedback loop for continuous assessment to help review and keep plans current	There was no evidence of strategic, tactical or operational-level strategic planning models found in this study in private or hospital pathology
Planning project and team structure	Jiang et al. (2002); Gray & Larson (2000)	Pre-planning partnering was implemented to look at IS planning and IS effectiveness success on the basis that the planning team is critical to project success and pre-planning partnering helps to remove potential conflicts	This research found that project planning, and consequently pre-planning partnering, did not to occur in pathology. The research found that there is an individual approach rather than a team approach to limited planning by individual stakeholders for the development of functional tools to aid in a specific, unique task. These developments were found to have no strategic value by this study
		Team structure and relationship of members is critical to project success and building a cohesive motivated team is a prelude to the accomplishment of project goals	This finding by the research shows an attitude of individualism that has no concept or interest in a team approach to planning and development of the pathology IS
		Top management should support the team structure and make finance available for the pre-planning partnering and team-building exercises	This research found that management did not support a team approach to planning in private or hospital pathology
Commoditisation of laboratory information systems	Friedberg (2008); Bossuyt et al. (2007)	Pathology information systems are regarded as a commodity and as such are not seen to have any strategic value— This compromises development of the pathology information systems as funds are not prioritised and made available for information systems development	
		Pathology information systems not viewed as a strategic tool due to lack of development and lack of technical capability. This compromises funding for development that further widens the technological void between pathology and other knowledge-based business verticals	

These key findings are instrumental in answering the primary research question "How does the effectiveness of laboratory information systems impact on business outcomes in medical pathology"? and the research sub-questions, "Does SISP occur in medical pathology in Australia" and "What are the determinants of information systems effectiveness in pathology laboratories in Australia"? These key findings and their impact and role in answering the research questions are discussed in detail below.

6.3.1   Commoditisation of Pathology Information Systems—Impact on Strategy

There is a strong view within the medical industry, both public and private sectors that the pathology information systems are a commodity and as such are not viewed as strategic. Hence the pathology information systems do not attract funds for development. The pathology information systems were shown not to have any strategic value *per se* and did not attract funds for strategic development. Contributing factors to the pathology information system being regarded as a commodity were found to have two major differences—in the hospital scenario, hospital management regarded pathology in general, and the pathology information system in particular, with a very low priority compared to other departments and services. The hospital pathology department was therefore at the bottom of the list when it came to the allocation of funds for development. Private pathology also lacked strategic funding of the laboratory as a whole, and specifically the pathology information system. This study found that there are two factors that contribute to lack of funds in private pathology—private pathology is regarded as a limited monopoly in Australia as there are only three major players. There is therefore little incentive for change as each player has a sizeable share of the market and is making good profits. The second contributing factor to lack of funding in private pathology in Australia is that all three major firms are public companies and therefore concentrate on maximising profits to enable the best possible shareholder returns.

The discussions in each of the three focus groups determined that the pathology information systems were regarded as a commodity and as such have no strategic value. This view in both private and hospital pathology largely determines funding. The hospital pathology laboratory is dependent on government funding, the amount of which relates to the priority in which top management within the hospital holds pathology, and the philosophy of the incumbent political party. Private pathology, a commercial operation, may have a scientific mission, but typically it is subordinated to economic considerations and considered success only in terms of net return on investment. Competition based only on price and financial considerations leads to commoditisation and often results in a race to the bottom of quality (Friedberg, 2008). The pathology information systems therefore attracted little capital for strategic development in both the hospital and private pathology settings in this study.

6.3.2   Pathology Information Systems Lack of Capability—Impact on Strategy and Business Outcomes

The research has also shown that mainframe pathology information systems are not scalable and flexible and are unable to support modern technology such as open architecture and client-server systems and this impacts negatively on business outcomes in both private and hospital pathology.

The data collected in all parts of this study have shown that both the hospital and private laboratory information systems lack the capability to support technological and strategic change. The survey data showed that pathology information systems capability is the influence on the process of strategic information systems planning and of information systems effectiveness. The ability for staff in pathology to undertake successful strategic planning was therefore primarily dependent on the pathology information systems being capable in its ability to support strategic planning itself. The survey data, however, showed that the survey participants did not agree that the pathology information systems are capable (Chap. 5), and this finding supports the earlier argument that lack of information system capability negatively impacts on business outcomes in pathology practice.

The pathology information systems were found to be functional rather than strategic in their use, which compounded their lack of scalability and flexibility. A distinction between information system functionality and capability was made in this research with respect to the pathology information systems in hospital and private pathology to assist in the determination of exactly what role the current pathology information systems play in strategic planning in pathology practice. In accordance with the Henderson and Venkatraman's (1999) Strategic Alignment Model (SAM), systemic capabilities can positively contribute to the creation of new business strategies, or better support the existing strategies. This research has shown that the pathology information systems in both hospital and private pathology lacked capability and that this has had a negative impact on business outcomes. The lack of capability of the studied pathology information systems thus affected the capacity of the organisations to establish effective strategic planning. This outcome supports the arguments of Rondeau et al. (2006); Hackney et al. (1999); Gerwin and Kolodny (1992); and Grover and Segars (2005) who argued that firms with high levels of organisational involvement in information systems-related activities have higher levels of information systems management effectiveness.

6.3.3   Lack of Use of Objective Means of Information Systems Effectiveness Measurement in Pathology

This research demonstrated that in the pathology laboratories studied there was no objective means for measuring and evaluating information systems planning effectiveness. The literature studied in this research has cited a number of methods of assessing information systems planning effectiveness, the commonly used methods being information system use, user information satisfaction (UIS) and decision support capability. UIS is the more favoured of these success measures, but remains controversial as UIS is regarded as behavioural/attitude phenomena and has little to do with the primary business goals of the firm (Grover and Segars 2005; Raghunathan and Raghunathan 1998; Lederer and Sethi 1998). The data analysis in this study into both private and hospital pathology showed there was recognition of UIS as an indicator of information systems effectiveness on an individual level for the functional tasks of the pathology information system. All participants agreed, however, that UIS was not a measure of strategic information systems effectiveness and concurred with the literature findings that UIS is unrelated to the business goals of the firm. In the context of the expansion into more modern business facilities, embracing service quality and e-commerce, for instance, both private and hospital pathology information systems are unable to support this expansion which embraces a service-centric approach. The means of measuring information systems effectiveness (Petter et al. 2008) in terms of service quality (SERVQUAL, for instance) is not able to be integrated into current mainframe pathology systems.

6.3.4 Strategic Information Systems Planning Was Not Evident in Pathology

This research has found that strategic planning activities previously mentioned in the research literature (Grover and Segars 2005; Grover et al. 1996; Rondeau et al. 2006; Petter et al. 2008) were not as evident in pathology practice in Australia in the exemplars used in this study. There are two important aspects of strategic planning that have been underemphasised, and this was found to be the case in this study in pathology practice in Australia. The first is the planning process or how planning is accomplished. The second is planning evolution or how planning evolves as a learning exercise (Grover and Segars 2005). Both perspectives can provide practical guidance on how organisations will change their planning process over time in an attempt to improve their effectiveness as well as leverage their investment in SISP. This research has shown that these planning activities were underemphasised in pathology practices to the detriment of business outcomes.

6.3.5 Financial Considerations, Business–IT and End-user Involvement and Their Impact on Planning

Financial issues relating to the pathology information systems and created by management in both private and hospital pathology were shown to have had a negative effect on pathology information systems effectiveness . Economic constraints within the healthcare system advocate the introduction of tighter control of costs. Based on cost information, proper decisions regarding priorities, procedure choices, personnel policies and investments can be made. This research has shown that hospital pathology has a low priority in the eyes of hospital management and as a result is not funded for development by the hospital management. Private pathology management has pressure and priority to maximise the return on investment to the investors, and as a consequence, funding for pathology information system development is not forthcoming.

Business–IT alignment and end-user involvement had a positive but small affect on strategic planning in the pathology practices studied. Business–IT alignment and end-user involvement in planning were not strong factors impacting on strategic planning in pathology practice in Australia. This research has shown that underlying this finding is a lack of understanding of the principles of strategic planning and their application and a lack of a cohesive approach to planning in pathology. Analysis of the research data pertaining to the FG1 and FG2 confirms that incremental development of pathology information systems is often an individual planning process, that is, a process for change is initiated by one person or one department. The participants in both focus groups gave examples of this approach and the examples demonstrated a lack of planning alignment and end-user involvement with the end result that the change initiated was not suited to the existing workflow systems. This research has further shown that due to lack of capability of the pathology information systems the alignment between business strategy and information systems was compromised. Grover and Segars (2005) argue that successful strategic planning of information systems should achieve alignment between the information systems and business strategy; should analyse and understand the business and associated technologies; should foster cooperation and partnership between managers and user groups; should anticipate relevant events/issues within the competitive environment and should adapt to unexpected organisational and environmental change. In this study of pathology information systems, both in the private and public sectors, there was little evidence of alignment between the information systems in use and business strategy; there was little evidence of all stakeholders being involved in analysis of either the business or the technologies in use; there was significant evidence that there was poor co-operation and almost no partnership between management and end users; and there was little evidence of co-operative change. Change was often forced.

The research into pathology practice in this study has shown that end-user involvement in the planning process does not occur significantly. The data collected in this study show that there is a gap in the individual needs of the scientists and the IT staff, and that there is a clear lack of communication with respect to pathology information systems development. This lack of communication often resulted in change and enhancement to the pathology information systems by the IT staff without consultation with the scientists to the detriment of the pathology workflow system. In an organisational context, this represented an inability for the pathology practices in this study to undertake any co-ordinated integration or any implementation of change and development.

Wang and Tai (2003) argued that contextual factors are important in strategic planning of information systems. They suggest that stakeholders not understanding context may lead to the planning system being less adaptable to different organisational contexts and therefore be overly deterministic. There was little evidence in either the public or private pathology of context planning. The lack of significant Business–IT alignment and end-user involvement in this study can be interpreted as undermining the planning system and information systems effectiveness that Wang and Tai (2003) alluded to, that is, commitment to planning, implementation mechanisms and acceptance of integration and planning mechanisms were compromised. These findings demonstrate that from the perspective of organisational and contextual considerations, hospital and private pathology practices in this study were lacking in an ability to undertake effective strategic planning.

The link between strategic planning and performance has been found to be inconsistent by Grover and Segars (2005) and Premkumar and King (1992). Some indicators suggested for assessment of information systems effectiveness have been information systems usage, UIS, quality of decision making, productivity from cost/benefit analysis and system quality (Ein-Dor and Segev 1978). The most commonly favoured factors have been information systems use and UIS. However, because of a lack of a theoretical framework for placing UIS within the greater context of overall "information systems effectiveness" its relevance as a performance measurement has been questioned (Grover and Segars 2005). This research has found that there was some recognition by the participants in the survey and in FG1 and FG2 that UIS, when applied to some functional data provision, was a satisfactory measure of information system effectiveness. This research also showed, however, that UIS as an acceptable measure of information system effectiveness was an individual view, and that UIS as a strategic measure of information system effectiveness was unacceptable to the scientists as end users. This view was supported by the research participants, who acknowledged that UIS has little, if any relevance to the business goals of the firm.

6.3.6 Service Quality in Pathology

The results of this research have shown that the effective use and further development of both hospital and private pathology information systems was compromised by the lack of attention by management given to the service quality in both the public and private sectors. The opportunity for the development of strategic plans involving the pathology information systems in an attempt to obtain a competitive advantage in the pathology industry was at best also compromised. This is attributable to the lack of capability of the existing pathology information systems to embrace modern technologies such as the internet, telemedicine and e-commerce shown by this research. The task-technology gap that is evident in pathology information systems has now expanded to include technical support for developing and efficient business trends that have a strong emphasis on service quality. This research has shown that existing pathology information systems are unable to accommodate such service quality analytical tools as SERVQUAL.

6.3.7   The Impact of a Monopoly in Private Pathology

The presence of a limited monopoly in private pathology, it can be argued, negatively influenced pathology information system development in private and hospital pathology in Australia. Private pathology practice in Australia consists of a limited monopoly of three publicly listed businesses. This research has demonstrated that the monopoly has had a two-fold impact on commoditisation of the pathology information systems in private pathology laboratories. The effects of the monopoly in private practice also impacted on those hospital laboratories that are managed and run by private pathology practices. Firstly, a monopoly tends to remove the need for development and innovation to achieve competitive advantage as a monopoly maintains an uncompetitive status quo. Secondly, and perhaps more dynamic in its impact on commoditisation and strategic spending, is that all three businesses in the monopoly are publicly listed and as such have a responsibility to their shareholders to maximise profit and stakeholder returns. For commercial pathology practice, the key drivers are economic. Industry requires a profit margin to appease the shareholder base and consequently must deliver services. Commercial operations may have a scientific mission, but typically it is subordinated to economic considerations and considered successful only if the net return is positive (Friedberg, 2008). This research has found that management decisions pertaining to laboratory equipment were based on cost analysis of reagents and had no strategic inferences. This determination by management also was shown to apply to the development of the pathology information systems. Spending was shown in this study to be functional and not strategic. To some extent this relates to the monopoly in private pathology practice in Australia.

6.3.8   Lack of Awareness of IT and Business Principles
in Management and IT Staff

Middle management was shown in this study not to be IT aware. The study also showed that the IT staff is not familiar with the business and strategic goals of the firms involved. This research has demonstrated that middle management in both private and hospital pathology is not aware of basic IT functionality and capability and this has been shown to have had a negative impact on any occurrence of pathology information systems development, and consequently on business outcomes. Middle management was not aware of more modern technologies such as open systems architecture and web-based systems. The ramifications of this lack of understanding have in the past compromised local development of the pathology information systems with the end result being a lack of pathology information system capability. As the private pathology practices have expanded internationally, this research has shown that the lack of awareness of middle management of modern IT capability restricted the practices' globalisation efforts in terms of modern capable and flexible IT support for pathology information systems effectiveness.

It has also been demonstrated by this research that the IT staff in both private and hospital pathology lack an understanding of business in general and the strategic goals of the practice in particular. This was especially evident in the focus group analysis where it was stated that the IT department would often make information system changes without any consultation with pathology staff as to what the changes were and how the changes would impact the business workflow and goals of the pathology laboratory. The research has also shown there to be the presence of bias and personal agendas within the management and IT staff that have been cited by participants of the focus groups as being major contras to an open and team-based approach to pathology information system development.

6.4 Summary

This research has investigated the level of strategic information systems planning in private and hospital pathology laboratories and its impact on business practice and development in pathology practice in Australia. The research also considered the role of two specific components introduced by the researcher relating to pathology laboratories, those being pathology information systems capability and the role of research and education in pathology information systems development and laboratory management.

The analysis of the data has shown that a lack end-user involvement and Business–IT alignment negatively impact on strategic planning in pathology practice, as they do in many other businesses. The data in this study have shown that pathology laboratory information systems capability is the dominant determinant of strategic planning in pathology laboratories in Australia. The participants in the study acknowledged that both the hospital and private pathology laboratory information systems are not capable and as a result of this, effective strategic planning is unlikely to be able to occur in both hospital and private pathology in Australia.

This research also found that, whilst financial considerations were acknowledged as being important in the management of the laboratory, financial considerations had no strategic role, that is, spending in private and hospital pathology laboratories in this study is functional and not strategic. This finding is in keeping with the work by Mayer (1998) on cost analysis in pathology and its impact on pathology development. He found also that the emphasis in pathology was one of cost containment at the expense of development, that is, that pathology analysers are no longer being selected for their quality and capacity. The cost per test was the only consideration used by the pathology in his study.

6.5 Conclusion

The research project was undertaken to investigate how the effectiveness of pathology information systems impacts on business outcomes in hospital and private pathology in Australia. The results of the research have shown that there is indeed a negative impact on business outcomes, principally based on the fact that the pathology information system is regarded as a commodity by those in the health vertical, and that the pathology information system lacks capability and fails in its ability to support the strategic development of the business. The negative attitude with which the various participants regard the pathology information systems illustrates that, in their view, it is not capable and it is therefore not a strategic tool.

Spending in private pathology was found to be functional and not strategic, in keeping with Friedberg's (2008) comments that commercial pathology laboratories may have a scientific mission, but typically it is subordinated to economic considerations and considered successful only if net return is positive. The alignment between the pathology scientists and IT staff was found to be lacking which further compromised efficiencies of planning and development. This is in contrast to the OpenLabs project in the UK (O'Moore et al. 1996; Boran et al. 1994) where the development of pathology was the focus of strategic planning and the key indicator of success and effectiveness.

The research, however, is limited in its ability to generate significant generalisations but does create the opportunity for further research that will enable more generalisations to be developed in the future. The key findings of this research have demonstrated not only that both private and hospital pathology are unable to use the principles of strategic information systems planning and apply them to information systems development but also that information systems effectiveness is not able to be measured in either the private or hospital pathology exemplars in this study. The research has also demonstrated that planning principles, when applied to pathology, do not fit with any recognised models cited in this research. The Henderson and Venkatraman's SAM, for example, has components of external strategy and internal capability in which the IT/information systems play a pivotal role. The lack of capability demonstrated by this research precluded the studied pathology information systems from achieving Business–IT alignment in the way suggested by the model.

This research has found that both private and hospital pathology information systems in the Australian exemplars used, through their lack of capability, scalability and flexibility, were unable to support the technologies required to enable the use of indicative success factors in modern business—e-commerce technologies, knowledge management systems and processes and the use of effective service quality measures such as the SERQUAL application (Petter et al., 2008; Delone and McLean 1995).

This research demonstrates that the pathology industry in Australia is lacking an organised and informed approach to strategic information systems planning, information system effectiveness measurement and the assessment of service quality. The technological void between pathology and other knowledge-based verticals could also be said to apply to business structure and existing planning processes.

6.6 Limitations of the Research

Throughout this study specific limitations were highlighted. The research design and methodology has limitations associated with this study being exploratory, the principal limitation being that, as an exploratory exercise, the methodology has no history of peer group review and acknowledgement of its validity as a research method. Despite a significant number of studies undertaken in other business verticals, this study breaks new ground and has had no established industry exemplar methodologies to follow.

The lack of sufficient responses to the survey instrument required a change in methodology to accommodate a lower sample number. In the original research methodology, structured equation modelling (SEM) was to be used as the pathway analysis technique. SEM requires a minimum sample number of approximately 250 samples for valid analysis results to be obtained (see Chap. 4—methodology). The survey provided only 96 completed questionnaires, which was clearly an insufficient number for SEM. After extensive evaluation of alternate methods of pathway analysis, which included partial least squares and linear multiple regression, linear multiple regression was deemed to be the most suitable and peer group ratified method to use. The novelty of this approach is a matter for caution until future research confirms (modifies or rejects) the findings by following a similar research paradigm.

The measuring instrument can bear some inherent limitations as it relies on one person's knowledge and ability to accurately convey their impressions into the questionnaire. Hence, the use of perceptual measures from a single respondent could result in potentially subjective judgements.

In some instances, the underlying assumptions in statistical methods can affect their validity and effectiveness. The lack of survey respondents was attributable to a lack of the Australian pathology industry's willingness to participate in this research project, and this presented limitations for the selection of quantitative methodology, as stated above. The relatively small number of respondents may potentially limit the diverse attitudes and opinions expressed by the population under study. The lack of willingness to participate also had an impact on the selection of the qualitative method that is, the lack of willingness to participate and the lack of time to participate contributed to the selection of focus groups and not individual interviews for this research. Also, the researcher's cognition and experience influence the result interpretation. The result presentation relies on the researcher alone, which could be a limiting factor due to the researcher's ability to communicate and present the complexity of research. The limitations associated with focus groups as used in this research are a lack of privacy that may influence respondents' comments and difficulties in recording the focus group and analyse the open-ended responses.

6.7 Future Research

Future research should address the limitations pertaining to the methodology used and the conduct of this research. The first and perhaps the most significant limitation, that being the lack of willingness of the industry to participate in this research project, needs to be overcome. This is a major problem and a means for persuading the pathology industry to participate in future research projects such as this work is unclear to the researcher. Perhaps an awareness by the pathology industry that there is active research now being undertaken in the vertical and that this research is making findings that will be beneficial to the vertical's business infrastructure and outcomes may allay some of the hesitancy and fears expressed by senior executives of pathology practice in this project. A larger number of participants and a willingness to participate would introduce more flexibility into the selection of research methodologies for future research i.e. SEM and one-on-one interviews would be available for use in methodologies of the future. The results obtained by a more extensive methodology base would serve to enrichen the research process and its outcomes through the achievement of a more confident level of generalisation.

Addressing the limitations found in this research would assist in obtaining an increased awareness of the pathology service in its rightful role as a consultancy service. This would contribute to pathology not being regarded as a commodity, which would result in a more favourable position for provision of funds for development and change in pathology in general.

6.7.1 Reverse SISP—A Developing Concept

Conventional SISP (Grover and Segars 2005; Grover et al. 1996; Petter et al. 2008) may be regarded as a planning exercise where the driver for change is initiated from within the business/firm, and may be driven by events such as:

1. A perceived advantage of an IT development to enhance business goal(s);
2. Solution to internal problems i.e. mainframe to open-architecture (OpenLabs);
3. Market research and interpretation of change in factors such as political and economic developments to get competitive advantage;
4. Economic and business factors.(Grover and Segars 2005; Grover et al. 1996)

The mechanism for conventional SISP involves such principles as Business–IT alignment, end-user involvement, pre-planning partnering and financial considerations (cost-benefit analysis) working together in a cohesive team effort to undertake to plan for, and execute, change (Grover and Segars 2005; Grover et al. 1996). This study has highlighted that an alternative perspective might be possible. Reverse SISP represents a demand on a participant of a vertical for change from other participants in that vertical. This change is in keeping with strategic developments of the vertical as a result of strategic pressure on the vertical. Reverse SISP is a situation whereby external factors and strategic pressure are brought to bear on the component of the vertical by other associated components of that vertical. The concept of reverse SISP arises from considerations of scenarios pertaining to hospital and private pathology as a result of external pressure, such as the implementation of the Healthsmart project, the State Government project for the implementation of a standardised IT platform for public health throughout Victoria. If other departments change, pathology will have to follow suit—the change in the other departments via Healthsmart will force it to. The decision to change will be out of the pathology's hands.

The concept of reverse SISP is based on change being initiated by external drivers for change, most likely from a closely related participant component of the same industry vertical. Reverse SISP results from considerable strategic pressure being placed on the vertical component lacking comparable technologies/business practices. In the case of the Healthsmart scenario, pathology is subject to external drivers to change, that is, other related hospital departments (radiology, cardiac catheter department). The drivers are that pathology is required to update its pathology information system to be able to accommodate the same ICT platform as the other departments and the hospital in general. There is a need to study the implications of reverse SISP in the application of the principles of SISP to other studies of pathology information systems and information systems in other verticals.

6.8   Implications of This Study for Practice and Research

The implications of the pathology information system being strategically incapable are both practical and academic. The practical implication is that the development and expansion of both hospital and private pathology in Australia is not supported by an efficient, modern IT platform. The ability to integrate modern ICT such as the internet, or even Web2, with voice over internet protocol (VOIP) telephony and intranets, for example, would provide more efficient information dissemination and co-operation amongst staff, especially when the international expansion of pathology in Australia is considered. This would enhance internal efficiencies that could lead to improved cost-effectiveness in the production of test results. The pathology information system would have the capacity to integrate with established technologies such as telemedicine and web-based voice recognition programs that would lend support to such strategic ventures as international expansion and the removal of workplace boundaries. The assessment of pathology information system effectiveness would be facilitated more objectively.

The ability to integrate the pathology information system with commercially available financial software packages could have sufficient positive impact to allow a change in business structure from a pyramidal hierarchy to a series of laterally linked self-funded business units. This could provide such management facilities as best practice and benchmarking, goal setting, and real-time cash flow, balance sheet and profit/loss statements that are currently unavailable.

The academic implication relates to assessing the effectiveness of the pathology information system. Without the ability to undertake strategic planning, there is little means of assessing information system effectiveness. This research has evolved a strategic planning information systems effectiveness model where the determinate for information system effectiveness is the attainment of a clearly established business goal that has been set after extensive analysis of the planned project and with the input of all relevant stakeholders. By way of publications relating to any effectiveness model, a more standardised approach to planning may evolve. This research has also highlighted the lack of formal education in pathology of strategic planning of pathology information systems and business in general, and discussions with course leaders following the findings of this research may lead to incorporation of strategic planning of pathology information systems and business principles into curriculum of future pathology practitioners.

The problem of solving the inefficiencies in both hospital and private pathology laboratories is widespread and complex. Firstly, there needs to be an awareness of the depth of the problem and this research will help in illuminating the general lack of ability for change. There needs to be a recognition that the systems (workflow and pathology information system) may not be as efficient as some people regard them. There needs to be a change in attitude towards the pathology information system in terms of priority for funding and recognition that the pathology information system may in fact be a strategic tool. The pathology information system may also be regarded as a critical component of a service-centric industry if it can be developed to be able to integrate with service quality measurement tools such as SERQUAL. The possible ways forward mentioned above could see large improvements made to this important aspect of healthcare and save a considerable amount of money, but any approach needs input and cooperation from all parties to be successful. Reading and research by all parties to understand the nuances of strategic planning of information systems is critical to the way forward; without this in place progress and development would suffer the same negative outcomes as seen in the pathology industry now.

Bossuyt et al. (2008) argue that pathology services should capitalise on the knowledge of the clinical staff and expand their business models to include service provision by way of clinical consultation to advise doctors on which test to order to best investigate the patients symptoms. Comments made by the participants of FG3 support Bossuyt et al.'s (2008) concept in the context of pathology being fundamental to the investigation of disease and that if services were improved by better alignment of tests requested with the disorder being investigated, pathology services could be delivered more effectively. The two possible benefits of this are a means of expanding a business that is seen in the eyes of most clients as a commodity with no strategic value, and a means to reduce the public cost of health by reducing the requesting of inappropriate blood tests. A study in the context of a change of attitude towards pathology in terms of pathology being viewed as an active consultancy service and what impact this would have on the commodity view and hence a more favourable provision of funds for development could provide the basis to initiate a change in the role of pathology services in general.

Finally, in closing we hope this book has served to open the door to more attention and research focus on the area of ICT use related to laboratory operations and pathology practices. An area that is of vital importance to effecting superior healthcare delivery.

References

Abdi, H. (2003). Encyclopaedia of Social Sciences Research Methods. M. Lewis-Beck, A. Bryman, & T. Futing (Eds.), Thousand Oaks: Sage.

Alter, S. I. (1992). *Information systems: A management perspective*. Reading: Addison-Wesley.

Anandarajan, M., & Arinze, B. (1998). Matching client/server processing architectures with information processing requirements: A contingency study. *Information and Management, 34,* 265–274.

Applegate, L. M., McFarlan, F. W., & McKenney, J. L. (1996). *Corporate information systems management: Text and cases.* Boston: Irwin/McGraw-Hill.

Avison, D., & Fitzgerald, G. (1995). *Information systems development: Methodologies, techniques and tools.* NY: McGraw-Hill.

Baets, W. (1992). Aligning information systems with business strategy. *The Journal of Strategic Information Systems, 1*(4), 205–213.

Baets, W. J. (1996). Some empirical evidence on IS strategy. Alignment in banking. *Information and Management, 30*(4), 155–177.

Bagozzi, R. (Ed.). (1994). *Principles of marketing research.* Oxford: Blackwell Publishers.

Bannister, F., & Remenyi, D. (2000). Acts of faith: Instinct, value and IT investment decisions. *Journal of Information Technology, 15,* 67–77.

Baroudi, J. J., & Orlikowski, W. J. (1988). A short-form measure of UIS: A psychometric evaluation and notes of use. *Journal of Management Information Systems, 4*(4), 44–59.

Barribeau, P., Butler, B., Corney, J., Doney, M., Gault, J., Gordon, J., Fetzer, R., Klein, A., Rogers, C. A., Stein, I. F., Steiner, C., Urschel, H., Waggoner, T., & Palmquist, M. (2005). Survey research, writing @ CSU, Colorado State University Department of English. Retrieved 27th September, 2008 from http://writing.colostate.edu/guides/research/survey.

Baskerville, R., & Lee, A. S. (1999). Distinctions among different types of generalizing in information systems research. In: L. Introna, M. Myres, & J. I. DeGross (Eds.), *Organisational processes: Field studies and theoretical reflection on the future of work* (pp. 49–65). New York: Klewer Academic.

Belkin, M., Corbitt, B., & Peszynski, K. (2008). *Multi-dimensional modelling in the health industry. Encyclopaedia of Healthcare Information Systems* (Vol. 111). New York: Hersey.

Bhattacherjee, A. (2001). Understanding information system continuance: An expectation-confirmation model. *MIS Quarterly, 25*(3), 351–370.

Blaikie, N. (2003). *Designing social research.* Cambridge: Polity Press, CB2 1UR.

Bokhari, R. H. (2005). The relationship between system usage and user satisfaction: A meta-analysis. *The Journal of Enterprise Information Management, 18*(2), 211–234.

M. Belkin et al., *Strategic ICT Planning in Pathology,*
Healthcare Delivery in the Information Age,
DOI 10.1007/978-1-4614-4478-7, © Springer Science+Business Media, LLC 2013

Boomsma, A. (1982). The robustness of LISREL Against Small Sample Sizes in Factor Analysis Models. In K. G. Joreskog & H. Wold (Eds.), *Systems under indirect observations, Part 1* (pp. 149–174). Amsterdam.

Boran, G., O'Moore, R., Grimson, W., Peters, M., Hasman, A., Groth, T., & Van Merode, F. (1996). A new clinical laboratory information system architecture from the OpenLabs project offering advanced services for laboratory staff and users. *Clinica Chimica Acta, 248,* 19–30.

Bossuyt, X., Verweire, K., & Blanckaert, N. (2007). Laboratory medicine: Challenges and opportunities. *Clinical Chemistry, 53*(10), 1730–1733.

Boynton, A. C., & Zmud, R. W. (1987). Information technology planning in the 1990's: Directions for practice and research. *MIS Quarterly, 11*(1), 58–71.

Brender, J., & McNair, P. (1996). User requirements on the future laboratory information systems. *Computer Methods and Programs in Biomedicine, 50,* 87–93.

Brender, J., Magdal, U., Wiegell, B., Schioler, T., & McNAir, P. (1993). Problem-oriented management of laboratory work through dynamic test scheduling. *Clinica Chimica Acta, 222,* 57–69.

Brewer, G. D. (1983). Assessing outcomes and effects. In K. S. Cameron & Whetten, D. A (Eds.), *Organisational effectiveness: A comparison of multiple models.* San Diego, Academic Press.

Broad, S. A. (1997). LIMS—A catalyst for re-engineering. *Laboratory Automation and Information Management, 33,* 9–12.

Bryman, A. (2004). Focus Groups. *Social Research Methods* (2nd Ed.). New York: Oxford University Press (Chapter 16).

Burn, J. M., & Szeto, C. (2000). A comparison of the views of business and IT management on success factors for strategic alignment. *Information and Management, 37*(4), 197–216.

Byrd, T. A., Lewis, B. R., & Bryan, R. W. (2006). The leveraging influence of strategic alignment on IT investment: An empirical examination. *Information and Management, 43,* 308–321.

Cameron, K. S., & Whetten, D. A. (1983). Organisational effectiveness: One model or several? In K. S. Cameron & D. A. Whetten (Eds.), *Organisational Effectiveness: A Comparison of Multiple Models.* San Diego: Academic Press.

Campbell, B. (2005). *Alignment: Resolving ambiguity within bounded choices.* PACIS, Bangkok, Thailand, 1–14.

Cerveny, R., & Clark, T. (1985). Conversations on Why information systems fail and what can be done about it. *Systems, Objectives, Solutions, 1,* 149–154.

Chan, Y. E., & Huff, S. L. (1993). Strategic information systems alignment. *Business Quarterly, 58*(1), 51–55.

Chan, Y. E., Huff, S. L., Barclay, D. G., & Copeland, D. G. (1997). Business strategic orientation, information systems strategic orientation and strategic alignment. *Information Systems Research, 8*(2), 125–150.

Chan, Y. E., & Reich, B. H. (2007). IT alignment: What have we learned? *Journal of Information Technology, 22,* 297–315.

Chi, G. (2005). *A study of developing loyalty model.* PhD thesis, Oklahoma State University.

Chin, W. W. (1998). The Partial Least Squares Approach for Structural Equation Modelling. In G. A. Marcoulides (Ed.), *Modern methods for business research* (pp. 295–336). Mahwah: Lawrence Erlbaum Associates.

Chin, W. W., & Newstead, P. R. (1999). Structural Equation Modelling Analysis in Small Samples Using Partial Least Squares. In R. H. Hoyle (Ed.), *Statistical strategies for small sample research* (pp. 307–341). Thousand Oaks: Sage.

Choe, J-M. (2003). The effect of environmental uncertainty and strategic applications of IS on a firm's performance. *Information and Management, 40,* 257–268.

Coakes, S. J. (2005). *SPSS: Analysis without anguish: Version 12.0 for Windows.* Australia: Wiley.

Connell, N. A. D., & Young, T. P. (2007). Evaluating healthcare information systems through an "enterprise" perspective. *Information and Management, 44,* 433–440.

Conrath, D. W., & Mignen, O. P. (1990). What is being done to measure user satisfaction with EDP/MIS. *Information and Management, 6,* 7–19.

Cook, T. D., & Campbell, D. T. (1978). The design and conduct of quasi-experiments and true experiments in field settings. In M. D. Dunnette (Ed.), *Handbook of industrial and organisational psychology* (pp. 223–326). Chicago: Rand McNally.

Coombs, C. R., Doherty, N. F., & Loan-Clarke, J. (2001). The importance of user ownership and positive user attitudes in the successful adoption of community information systems. *Journal of End User Computing, 13*(4), 5–16.

Cowan, C., Gray, C., & Larson, E. (1992). Project partnering. *Project Management Journal, 22*(4), 5–11.

Cresswell, J. (2003). *Research design—Qualitative, quantitative and mixed methods approaches* (2nd ed.). Thousand Oakes: Sage.

Cron, W. L., & Sobal, M. G. (1983). The relationship between computerisation and performance; a strategy for maximising the economic benefits for computerisation. *Information and Management, 6,* 171–181.

Cudeck, R., & Hensly, S. J. (1991). Model selection in covariance structure analysis and the 'Problem' of sample size: A clarification. *Psychological Bulletin, 109,* 512–519.

Davern, M., & Kauffman, R. (2000). Discovering potential and realising value from information technology investments. *Journal of Management Information Systems, 16*(4), 69–78.

Davis, F. D. (1989). Perceived usefulness, perceived ease of use, and user acceptance of information technology. *MIS Quarterly, 13*(3), 319–339.

Davis, G. B., & Olson, M. H. (1985). *Management information systems*. New York: McGraw Hill.

De Leede, J., Looise, J. C., & Alders, B. (2002). Innovation, improvement and operations: An exploration of the management of alignment. *International Journal of Technology Management, 23*(4), 353–368.

DeLone, W., & McLean, E. R. (2003). The DeLone and McLean model of information systems success: A ten year update. *Journal of Management Information Systems, 19*(4), 9–30.

DeLone, W. H., & McLean, R. E. (1992). Information systems success: The quest for the dependent variable. *Information Systems Research, 3*(1), 60–95.

DeLone, W. H., & McLean, E. R. (2004). Measuring e-commerce success: Applying DeLone and McLean information systems success model. *International Journal of Electronic Commerce, 9*(1), 31–47.

DOH. (1997). *The new NHS: Modern. Dependable*. London: HMSO.

DOH. (2002). *Delivering the 21st century IT support for the NHS: National strategic programme*. London: HMSO.

Doll, W. J. (1985). Avenues for top management involvement in successful MIS development. *MIS Quarterly, 9*(1), 17–35.

Doll, W. J., Xia, W., & Torkzadeh, G. (1994). A confirmatory factor analysis of the end-user computing satisfaction instrument. *MIS Quarterly, 18*(4), 453–461.

Dooley, L. M. (2002). *Advances in developing human resources*. Thousand Oakes: Sage.

Earl, M. J. (1993). Experiences in strategic information systems planning. *MIS Quarterly, 17*(1), 1–24.

Ein-Dor, P., & Segev, E. (1978). Organisational context and the success of MIS. *MIS Quarterly, 24*(10), 1–24.

Eisenhardt, K. M. (1989). Making fast strategic decisions in high velocity environments. *Academy of Management Journal, 32*(3), 543–576.

Falk, R. F., & Miller, N. B. (1992). *A primer of soft modelling*. Akron: The University of Akron Press.

Farbey, B., Land, F., & Targett, D. (1999). The moving staircase: Problems of appraisal and evaluation in a turbulent environment. *Information Technology and People, 12*(3), 238–252.

Fishbein, M. (1967). Attitude and the prediction of behaviour. In M. Fishbein (Ed.), *Reading in attitude theory and measurement* (pp. 477–492). New York: Willey.

Fishbein, M., & Ajzen, I. (1975). *Belief, Attitude, Intention and Behaviour: An Introduction to Theory and Research*, Reading: Addison-Wesley.

Flaval, D. J., & Williams, J. (1996). *Strategic Management*. New York: Prentice Hall.

Fornell, C., & Larcker, D. F. (1981). *Outsourcing information technology: Contracts and the client/vendor relationship.* Oxford: Templeton College.

Frank, I. E., & Friedman, J. H. (1993). A statistical view of chemometrics regression tools. *Technometrics, 35,* 109–148.

Fredrickson, J. W. (1984). The comprehensiveness of strategic decision processes: Extension, observations, future directions. *Academy of Management Journal, 27*(3), 445–466.

Friedberg, R. C. (2008). Time for a reality check. A hospital-based laboratory's perspective. *Archives of Pathology & Laboratory Medicine, 132,* 781–784.

Friedman, B. (2005). What's ailing pathology: Why informatics will provide strong medicine. https://www.labinfotech.org/LIS2006/Presentations2005/Friedman_las_vegas_200 cited 18/9/2006.

Gallies, R. D. (1991). Strategic information systems planning: Myths, reality and guidelines for successful implementation. *European Journal of Information Systems, 1*(1), 55–64.

Gallies, R. D., & Samogyi, S. K. (1987). *From data processing to strategic information systems—a historical perspective, in towards strategic information systems.* London: Abacus Press.

Garson, D. (Copyright 1998, 2007– accessed 16th June, 2006), www2.chass.ncsu.edu/garson/pa765/factor/htm

Gation, A. W. (1994). Is user satisfaction a valid measure of system effectiveness? *Information and Management, 26,* 119–131.

Gerwin, D., & Kolodny, H. (1992). *Management of advanced manufacturing technology: Strategy, organisations and innovation.* New York: Wiley.

Gibbs, A. (1997). *Social research update 19.* UK: University of Surrey.

Glynn, C. J., Herbst, S., O'Keefe, G. J., Shipiro, R. Y., & Lindeman, M. (2004). *Public opinion.* Boulder: Westview Press, p. 312.

Goldschmidt, H. M. J., de Vries, J. C. M., van Merode, G. G., & Derks, J. J. M. (1998). A workflow management tool for laboratory medicine. *Laboratory Automation and Information Management, 33,* 183–197.

Goodhue, D., Lewis, W., & Thompson, R. (2006). PLS, Small Sample Size and Statistical Power in MIS Research. In *Proceedings of the 39th Hawii International Conference on Social Sciences,* R. Sprague Jr. (Ed.), Kaurii, Hawaii.

Gorla, N. (1989). Identifying MIS research issues using a research framework. *Information and Management, 17,* 131–141.

Gray, C. F., & Larsom, E. W. (2000). *PROJECT management: The managerial process.* Boston: Irwin, McGarw-Hill.

Greiner, L. E. (1972). Evolution and revolution as organisations grow. *Harvard Business Review, 50*(4), 37–46.

Grover, V, & Segars, A. H. (2005). An empirical evaluation of stages of strategic information systems planning: Patterns of process design and effectiveness. *Information and Management, 42,* 761–799.

Grover, V., Jeong, S. R., & Segars, A. H. (1996). Information systems effectiveness: The construct space and patterns of application. *Information and management, 31,* 177–191.

Grover, V., Teng, J., Segars, A. H., & Fielder, K. (1998). The influence of information technology diffusion and business process change on perceived productivity: The IS executives perspective, *Information and Management, 34,* 215–221.

Gummesson, E. (1991). *Qualitative Methods in Management Research.* London: Sage.

Hackney, R., Kawalek, J., & Dhillon, G. (1999). Startegic information systems planning: Perspectives on the role of the end-user revisited. *Journal of end-user computing, 11*(2), 3–12.

Hair, J. F., Anderson, R. E., Tatham, R. L., & Black, W. C. (1998). *Multivariate data analysis* (5th ed.). Upper Saddle River: Prentice-Hall International Inc.

Hair, J, Black, W, Babin, B, Anderson, R., & Tatham, R. (2006). *Multivariate Data Analysis* (6th ed.). New Jersey: Prentice-Hall.

Hamilton, S., & Chervany, N. L. (1981). Evaluating information system effectiveness—Part 1: Comparing evaluating approach. *MIS Quarterly, 5*(4), 79–86.

Helland, I. S. (1990). PLS regression and statistical methods. *Scandinavian Journal of Statistics, 17,* 97–114.

Henderson, J. C., & Sifonis, J. G. (1988). The value of strategic IS planning: Understanding consistency, validity and IS markets. *MIS Quarterly, 12*(2), 187–200.

Henderson, J. C., & Venkatraman, N. (1993). Strategic alignment leveraging information technology for transforming organisations, *IBM Systems Journal, 32*(1).

Henderson, J. C., Rockart, J. F., & Sifonis, J. G. (1987). Integrating management support systems into strategic information systems planning. *Journal of Management Information Systems, 4*(1), 3–14.

Hines, T. (1998). *Management information for marketing and sales.* Oxford: Butterworth-Heinemann.

Hines, T. (2000). An evaluation of two qualitiative methods (focus group interviews and cognitive maps) for conducting research into entrepreneurial decision making. *Qualitative Market Research: An International Journal, 3*(1), 7–16.

Hirscheim, R., & Smithson, S. (1986). A critical analysis of information systems evaluation, Research and discussion paper—RDP 86/13, Oxford Institute of Information Management.

Horngren, C. T., & Foster, G. (1991). *Cost accounting. A managerial emphasis.* (7th ed.). New Jersey: Prentice Hall.

Hoskuldson, A. (1988). PLS regression methods. *Journal of Chemometrics, 2,* 211–228.

Hoyle, R. Ed. (1995). *Structural equation modelling: Concepts, issues and applications.* Thousand Oaks: Sage. (An introduction focusing on AMOS).

IBM Corporation (1981). Business systems planning—information systems planning guide, GE20-0527-3.

Irani, Z. (2002). Information systems evaluation: Navigating through the problem domain. *Information Management, 419,* 11–24.

Irani, Z., & Love, P. E. D. (2001). Information systems evaluation: past, present and future. *European Journal of information Systems, 10,* 183–188.

Irani, Z., & Love, P. E. D. (2002). Developing a frame of reference for ex-ante IT/IS investment evaluation. *European Journal of Information Systems, 11*

Ives, B., Olson, M. H., & Baroudi, J. J. (1983). The measurement of user information satisfaction. *Communications of the ACM, 26*(10), 785–793.

Jackson, D. L. (2003). Revisiting Sample Size and the Number of Parameter Estimates: Some Support for the N:q Hypothesis. *Structural Equation Modelling, 10,* 128–141.

Janesick, V. J. (2000). The choreography of qualitative research designs; minuets, improvisations and crystallisation. In N. K. Denzin & Y. S. Lincoln (Eds.), *Handbook of qualitative research,* (2nd ed., p. 379–400). Thousand Oaks: Sage.

Jennex, M. E., & Olfman, L. (2002). Organisational memory/knowledge effects on productivity: A longitudinal study. In *proceeding of the Thirty-Fifth Hawaii International Conference on Systems Sciences* (Sprague Jr, R. H, Ed.), p.109, IEEE Computer Society Press, Big Island, Hawaii, USA.

Jiang, J. J., Klein, G., & Discenza, R. (2002). Pre-project partnering impact on an information system project, project team and project manager. *European Journal of Information Systems, 11,* 86–97.

Johnson, R. B., & Onwuegbuzie, A. J. (2004). Mixed methods research: A research paradigm whose time has come. *Educational Researcher, 33*(7), 14–26.

Kahneman, D., Slovic, P., & Tversky, A. (1982). *Judgement under uncertainty: Heuristics and biases.* Chichester: Cambridge University Press.

Kaplan, B. (1987). The medical computing 'lag': perceptions of barriers to the application of computers to medicine. *International Journal of Assessment Health Care, 3*(1), 123–126.

Kearns, G. S., & Lederer, A. L. (2000). The effect of strategic alignment on the use of IS-based resources for competitive advantage. *Journal of Strategic Information Systems, 9*(4), 265–293.

Kearns, G. S., & Lederer, A. L. (2003). A resource-based view of strategic IT alignment: How knowledge sharing creates competitive advantage. *Decision Sciences, 34*(1), 1–29.

Kidder, L. H., & Judd, C. M. (1986). *Research Methods in Social Relations* (5th ed.). New York, Holt, Rinehart and Winston.

King, W. R. (1988). How effective is your information system planning? *Long Range Planning, 21*(5), 103–112.

Kitzinger, J. (1995). BMJ Education and Debate Series: Qualitative research; introducing focus groups. http://www.bmj.com/cgi/content/full/311/7000/299

Kivijarvi, H., & Saarinen, T. (1995). Investment in information systems and the financial performance of the firm. *Information and Management, 28,* 143–163.

Klecun, E., & Cornford, T. (2005). A critical approach to evaluation. *European Journal of Information Systems, 14,* 229–243.

Kline, P. (1994). *An Easy Guide to Factor Analysis.* London and New York: Routledge.

Krieg, A. F., Israel, M., Fink, R., & Shearer, L. K. (1978). A approach to cost analysis of clinical laboratory services. *American Journal of Clinical Pathology, 69,* 525–536.

Kulkarni, U. R., Ravindran, S., & Freeze, R. (2006). A knowledge management success model: Theoretical development and empirical validation. *Journal of management Information Systems, 23*(3), 309–347.

Larson, E. (1997). Partnering on construction projects: A study of the relationship between partnering activities and project success. *IEEE Transactions on Engineering Management, 44*(2), 188–195.

Laudon, K. C., & Laudon, J. P. (1991). *Management Information Systems: A Contemporary Perspective,* (2nd ed.). New York: MacMillan.

Le Blanc, L. A. (1991). SOS: An assessment of DSS performance. *Information and Management, 20,* 137–148.

Lederer, A. L., & Sethi, V. (1996). Key prescriptions for strategic information systems planning. *Journal of Management Information Systems,* 13(1), 35–62.

Lederer, A. L., & Sethi, V. (1998). The implementation of strategic information system planning methodologies. *MIS Quarterly, 12*(3), 444–461.

Levy, D. L. (2000). Applications and limitations of complexity theory in organisation theory and strategy. In J. Rabin, G. J. Miller, & W. B. Hildreth (Eds.), *Handbook of Strategic Management* (2nd edn., pp. 67–87). New York: Marcel.

Li, M., & Ye, L. R. (1999). Information technology and firm performance: Linking with environment, strategic and managerial contexts. *Information and Management, 35,* 43–51.

Linberg, K. R. (1999). Software developer perceptions about software project failure: A case study. *The Journal of Systems and Software, 49*(2/3), 177–192.

Lincoln, T. (1986). Do computer systems really pay off? *Information and Management, 11,* 25–34.

Lincoln, T. J. (1976). *The Future Constraints,* The Oxford Centre for Management Studies Top Management Briefing report.

Lincoln, T. J. (1980). *Information System Constraints—A Strategic Review,* IFIP Congress.

Lincoln, Y. S., & Guba, E. G. (1985). *Naturalistic Inquiry.* Beverley Hills: Sage.

Loehlin, J. C. (1992). *Latent variable models: An introduction to factor, path and structural analysis,* (2nd Ed.). Hillsdale: Lawrence Erlbaum.

Lucas, H. C. (1981). *Implementation—the key to successful information systems.* NY: Columbia University Press.

Luftman, J., Kempaiah, R., & Nash, E. (2005). Key issues for IT executives 2005. *MIS Quarterly Executive, 5*(2), 81–101.

Lyytinen, K. (1987). A taxonomic perspective of information system development: Theoretical constructs and recommendations. In R. J. Boland & R. A. Hirschheim (Eds.), *Critical issues in information systems research* (pp. 3–41). New York: Wiley.

MacCallum, R. C., Browne, M. W., & Sugawara, H. M. (1996). Power Analysis and Determination of Sample Size for Covariance Structure Modelling. *Psychological Methods, 1,* 130–149.

Magal, S. R., Carr, H. H., & Watson, H. J. (1988). Critical success factors for information centre managers. *MIS Quarterly, 12*(3), 412–425.

Mahmood, M. A., Hall, L., & Swanberg, D. L. (2001). Factors affecting information technology use: A meta-analysis of the empirical literature. *Journal of Organisational Computing and Electronic Commerce, 11*(2), 107–130.

March, I. G., & Simon, H. A. (1963). *Organisations.* New York, Wiley.

Marcoulides, G. A., & Saunders, C. (2006). PLS: A silver bullet? *MIS Quarterly, 30*(2), 3–9.

Mason, R. O. (1978). Measuring information output: A communication systems approach. *Information and Management, 1*(5), 219–234.

Mayer, M. (1998). Laboratory cost control and financial management software. *Clinica Chimica Acta, 270,* 55–64.

McBride, N. (1998). Towards a dynamic theory of information systems planning in *Proceeding of the 3rd UKAIS Conference,* Lincoln University, 218–230.

McKay, J., & Marshall, P. (2001). The IT evaluation and benefits management life cycle. In W. V. Grembergen (Ed.), *Information technology evaluation methods and management* (pp. 44–56). London: Idea Group Publishing.

McLean, E. R., & Soden, J. V. (1977). *Strategic planning for MIS.* New York: Wiley.

Menachemi, N., Saunders, C., Chukmaitov, A., & Matthews, M. C. (2007). Hospital adoption of information technologies and improved patient safety: A study of 98 hospitals in Florida. *Journal of Healthcare Management, 52*(6), 398–411.

Merton, R. (1987). The focuses interview and focus groups: Continuities and discontinuities. *Public Opinion Quarterly, 51,* 550–566.

Miller, J., & Doyle, B. A. (2001). Measuring the effectiveness of computer-based information systems in the financial services sector, *MIS quarterly, March,* 107–124.

Mingers, J. (2001). Combining IS research methods—towards a pluralist methodology. *Information Systems Research, 12*(3), 240–259.

Moad, J. (1989). Asking users to judge IS. *Datamation, 3*(21), 93–100.

Molla, A., & Licker, P. S. (2001). E-commerce systems success: An attempt to extend and respecify the DeLone and McLean model of IS success. *Journal of Electronic Commerce Research, 2*(4), 131–141.

Morgan, D. L. (1997). *Focus groups as qualitative research* (2nd Ed.). London: Sage.

Morse, J. (1991). On the evaluation of qualitative proposals. *Qualitative Health Research, 1*(2), 147–151.

Mumford, E., Hirschheim, R., Fitzgerald, G., & Wood-Harper, T. (1985). *Research methods in information. systems.* North Holland, Elsevier.

Neuman, W. L. (2003). *Social research methods: Quantitative and qualitative approaches.* New York: Pearson Education, Inc.

Nolan, R. L. (1979). Managing the crises in data processing. *Harvard Business review, 57*(2), 115–126.

Nunnally, J. C. (1978). *Psychometric theory* (2nd ed.). New York: McGraw-Hill.

Nunnally, J. C., & Bernstein, I. H. (1994). *Psychometric theory* (3rd ed.). New York: McGraw-Hill.

O'Brien, K. (1993). Improving survey questionnaires through focus groups. In D. Morgan (Ed.), *Successful focus groups: Advancing the state of the art* (pp. 105–118). London: Sage.

O'Moore, R. R., De Moor, G., Boran, G., Gaffney, P., Grimson, J., McNair, P., Groth, T., Nykanen, P., Eller, J., Yearworth, M., Willems, J., Brender, J., Scott, P., Schilders, L., Clarke, B., Peters, M., Grimson, W., & McAllister, B. (1994). OpenLabs: The application of advanced informatics and telematics for optimisation of clinical laboratory services. *Computer Methods and Progress in Biomedicine, 45,* 137–140.

Parasuraman, A. (1988). SERVQUAL: A multi-item scale for measuring customer perceptions of service quality. *Journal of Retailing, 64*(1), 12–40.

Parasuraman, A. (1991). Refinement of reassessment of the SERVQUAL scale. *Journal of Retailing, 67*(4), 420.

Parasuraman, A. (1993). Research note: More on the improving service quality measurement. *Journal of Retailing, 69*(1), 140.

Parasuraman, A. (1994). Reassessment of expectations as a comparison standard in measuring service quality—implications. *Journal of Marketing, 58*(1), 111.

Parasuraman, A., Zeithaml, V. A., & Berry, L. L. (1985). A conceptual model of service quality and its implications for future research. *Journal of Marketing, 49*(Fall), 41–50.

Peters, T. (1999). The WOW project. *Fast Company, 24*, 118–134.

Peters, T., & Homer, J. (1996). Learning to lead, to create quality, to influence change in projects. *Project Management Journal, 27*(1), 5–11.

Petter, S., DeLone, W., & McLean, E. (2008). Measuring information systems success: Models, dimensions, measures, and interrelationships. *European Journal of Information Systems, 17*, 236–263.

Pitt, L. F., Watson, R. T., & Kavan, C. B. (2001). Service quality: A measure of information systems effectiveness. *MIS Quarterly, June*, 173–187.

Prekumar, G., & King, W. R. (1992). An empirical assessment of information systems planning and the role of information systems in organisations. *Journal of Management Information Systems, 9*(2), 99–125.

Porter, M. E., & Millar, V. E. (1985). How information gives you competitive advantage. *Harvard Business Review, 63*(4), 149–160.

Porter, M. E., & Olmsted Teisberg, E. (2004). Redefining competition in health care. *Harvard Business Review, 82*(64), 64–76.

Powney, J. (1988). Structured eavesdropping. *Research Intelligence: Journal of the British Educational Research Foundation, 28*, 10–12.

Pyburn, P. J. (1983). Linking the MIS plan with corporate strategy: An exploratory study. *MIS Quarterly, 7*(2), 1–14.

Raghunathan, B., & Raghunathan, T. S. (1988). Impact of top management support on IS planning. *Journal of Information Systems, 2*(2), 15–23.

Ragowsky, A., Ahituv, N., & Neuman, S. (1996). Identifying the value of importance of an information system application. *Information and Management, 31*, 89–102.

Rai, A., Lang, S. S., & Welker, R. B. (2002). Assessing the validity of IS success models: An empirical test and theoretical analysis, *Information Systems Research, 13*(1), 5–69.

Ramamijan, V., & Venkatraman, N. (1987). Planning system characteristics and planning effectiveness. *Strategic Management Journal, 8*(5), 453–468.

Reich, B. H., & Benbasat, I. (2000). Factors that influence the social dimension of alignment between business and information technology objectives. *MIS Quarterly, 24*(1), 81–113.

Reich, B. H., & Benbasat, I. (2003). Measuring the information systems—business strategy relationship. In R. D. Galliers & D. E. Leidner (Eds.), *Strategic information management—challenges and strategies in managing information systems*. Oxford: Butterworth Heinemann.

Remenyi, D., Williams, B., Money, A., & Swatz, E. (1998). *Doing research in business and management—an introduction to process and methods*. London: Sage.

Renkema, T. J. W., & Berghout, E. W. (1997). Methodologies for information-systems investment evaluation at the proposal stage—a comparative review. *Information and Software Technology, 39*, 1–13.

Revere, L., & Roberts, R. (2004). Improving resource efficiency through management science. *Journal of Healthcare Management, 49*(5), 324–335.

Rondeau, P. J., Ragu-Nathan, T. S, & Vonderembse, M. A. (2006). How involvement, IS management effectiveness, and end-used computing impact IS performance in manufacturing firms. *Information and Management, 43*, 93–107.

Rubin, H. (2004). Into the light. In *CIO Magazine*. http://www.cio.com.au/index.php/id; 1718970659, accessed on July, 2004.

Rushinek, A., & Rushinek, S. F. (1986). What makes users happy? *Communications of the ACM, 29*(7), 594–598.

Saarinen, T. (1996). An expanded instrument for evaluating information system success. *Information and Management, 31*, 103–118.

Sabherwal, R., & King, W. R. (1995). An empirical taxonomy of the decision making process concerning strategic applications of information systems. *Journal of Management Information Systems, 11*(4), 177–214.

Sabherwal, R., Jeyaraj, A., & Chowa, C. (2006). Information systems success: individual and organisational determinants. *Management Science, 52*(12), 1849–1864.

Sambamurthy, V., Venkatraman, S., & Desanctis, G. (1993). The design of information technology planning systems for varying organisational contexts. *European Journal of Information Systems, 2910*, 23–35.

Sarantakos, S. (2005). *Social Research* (3rd ed.). New York: Palgrave Macmillan.

Schwalbe, K. (2000). *Information technology project management*. Cambridge: Course Technology.

Seddon, P., & Yip, S-K. (1992). An empirical evaluation of user information satisfaction (UIS) measures for use with general ledger accounting software. *Journal of Information Systems, 6*(1), 75–98.

Seddon, P., Graeser, V., & Willcocks, L. (2002). Measuring organisational IS effectiveness: An overview and update of senior management perspectives. *The Data Base for Advances in Information Systems, 33*(2), 11–28.

Sedera, D., Gable, G., & Chan, T. (2004). A factor and structural equation analysis of the enterprise systems success measurement model. In *Proceeding of the Twenty-Fifth International Conference on Information Systems* (Applegate, L., Galliers, R., & DeGross, J. I., Eds) p. 449, Association for Information Systems, Washington, DC, USA.

Segars, A. H. (1997). Assessing the unidimensionality of measurement: A paradigm and illustration within the context of information systems research. *Omega, 25*(1), 107–121.

Segars, A. H., & Grover, V. (1998). Strategic information systems planning success: An investigation of the construct and its measurement. *MIS Quarterly, 22*(2), 139–163.

Singh, S. K. (1993). Using information technology effectively. *Information & Management, 24*, 133–146.

Smithson, S., & Hirschheim, R. (1998). Analysing information systems evaluation: Another look at an old problem. *European Journal of Information Systems, 7*, 158–174.

Steiner, G. A. (1979). *Strategic planning: What every manager must know*. New York: Free Press.

Strassman, P. A. (1984). Information technology and productivity. *PITCOM, 3*(1), 1–19.

Strauss, A., & Corbin, J. (1998). *Basics of qualitative research: Techniques and procedures for developing grounded theory*. Thousand Oaks: Sage.

Srinivasan, A. (1985). Alternative measures of system effectiveness: Association and involvement. *MIS Quarterly, 9*(3), 243–253.

Stockberger, D. W. Correlation: Introductory Statistics: Concepts, Models, and Applications. http://business.clayton.edu?arjomand/book/sbk17.htm (Accessed 9th August, 2007).

Sugumaran, V., & Arogyaswamy, B. (2004). Measuring IT performance: "Contingency" variables and value modes. *The Journal of Computer Information Systems, 44*(2), 79–86.

Sullivan, C. H., Jr. (1985). Systems planning in the information age. *Sloan Management Review, 26*(2), 3–12.

Symons, V. J. (1991). A review of information systems evaluation: Content, context and process. *European Journal of Information Systems, 1*(3), 205–212.

Tallon, P., Kraemer, K., & Gurbaxani, V. (2000). Executives perceptions of the business value of information technology: A process-orientated approach. *Journal of Management Information Systems, 33*(2), 145–173.

Tashakkori, A., & Teddlie, C. (2003). *Handbook of mixed methods in social and behavioural research*. Thousand Oaks: Sage.

Teddlie, C., & Tashakkori, A. (2006). *A general typology of research designs featuring mixed methods. Research in the Schools, 13*(1), p.12.

Tenenhaus, M. (1998). *La regression PLS*. Paris: Technip.

Teubner, R. A. (2007). Strategic information systems planning: A case study from the financial services industry. *Journal of Strategic Information Systems, 16*, 105–125.

Thurstone, L. L. (1935). *The Vectors of Mind*. Chicago: University of Chicago Press.

Thurstone, L. L. (1947). *Multiple factor analysis: A development and expansion of the vectors of mind*. Chicago: University of Chicago Press.

Torke, N., Boral, L., Nguyen, T., Perri, A., & Chakrin, A. (2005). Process improvement and operational efficiency through test result autoverification. *Clin. Chem, 51*, 2406–2408.

Trice, A. W., & Treacy, M. E. (1986). Utilisation as a dependent variable in MIS research, *Proceeding of the 7th ICIS*, 227–239.

Van Merode, G. G., Hasman, A., Derks, J., Schoenmaker, B., & Goldschmidt, H. M. J. (1996). Advanced management facilities for clinical laboratories. *Computer Methods and Programs in Biomedicine, 50*, 195–205.

Venkatraman, N. & Ramanujaman, V. (1987). Planning system success: A conceptualisation and an operational model. *Management Science, 33*(6), 687–714.

Walsham, G. (1993). *Interpreting information systems in organisations*. Chichester:Wiley.

Wang, E. T. C. & Tai, J. C. F. (2003). Factors affecting information systems planning effectiveness: Organisational contexts and planning systems dimensions. *Information and Management, 40*, 287–303.

Weill, P., & Olson, M. H. (1989a). An assessment of the contingency theory of management information systems. *Journal of MIS, 6*(1), 59–85.

Weill, P., & Olsen, M. H. (1989b). Managing investments in information technology mini-case examples and implications. *MIS Quarterly, 13*, 3–17.

Wells, I. G., Farnan, L. P., & Rayment, M. W. (1996). Client/server computing: Is this the future direction for the clinical laboratory? *Clinica Chimica Acta, 248*, 31–38.

Wickramasinghe, N., Bali, R. Lehaney, B., & Gibbons, C. (2009). *HCKM Primer*. New Jersey: Routledge

Wilcocks, L. (2000). Evaluating the outcomes of information systems plans—managing information technology evaluating technologies and processes. In R. D. Galliers, D. E. Leidner, & B. S. H. Baker (Eds.), *Strategic information management—challenges and strategy in managing information systems*. Oxford: Butterworth Heinemann.

Yap, C. S., & Walsham, G. (1986). A survey of information technology in the UK service sector. *Information and Management, 10*(5), 267–274.

Youthas, K., & Young, S. T. (1998). Material matters: Assessing the effectiveness of materials management IS. *Information and Management, 33*, 115–124.

Zeithaml, V. A., Berry, L. L, & Parasuraman, A. (1993). The nature and determinants of customer expectations of service. *Journal of the Academy of Marketing Science, 21*(1), 1–12.

Zhu, K., & Kraemer, K. L. (2005). Post-adoption variations in usage and value of e-business by organisations: cross-country evidence from the retail industry. *Information Systems Research, 16*(1), 61–84.

Zikmund, W. G. (1997). *Business research methods*. New York: The Dryden Press Harcourt Brace College Publishers.

Zmud, R. W., Boynton, A. C, & Jacobs, G. C. (1986). The information economy: A new perspective for effective information systems management. *Database, 18*(1), 17–23.

Zinn, J., Zalokowski, A., & Hunter, L. (2001). Identifying indicators of laboratory management performance: A multiple constituency approach. *Health Care Management Review, 26*(1), 40–53.

Index

A
Application specialists, 72
ASP model, 77

B
Business goals, 7, 8, 14, 23, 33, 101, 103
Business-IT alignment, 3, 5, 37, 40, 41, 43, 44, 52, 58, 65, 72, 73, 77–79, 84, 102, 106, 108
Business outcomes, 3–5, 48, 51, 68, 79, 86, 88, 89, 91, 92, 101, 104

C
CCU, 66, 76
Close-knit team, 5
Composite planning models, 32, 37
Computer-based information systems (CBIS), 30

D
Decision making quality, 15, 103
Decision-makers problems, 11
Decision-making goals, 16
Diagnostic services, 1

E
Effective system, 5, 15, 22
Empirical research, 33
End-user involvement, 3, 5, 7, 20, 21, 37, 38, 43, 44, 52, 58, 77, 79, 102, 108
EUCS instrument, 23, 37

F
Financial considerations, 3, 53, 56, 58, 61, 70, 79, 84, 99, 101, 108
Frustration, 76
Future research, 36, 58, 89, 107, 108

H
Haematology analyser, 64
Hospital laboratory, 4, 46, 58, 66, 68, 72, 76, 82

I
IBM, 41
ICU, 66, 76
Information systems effectiveness, 15–23, 26, 29–31, 35, 37–39, 43, 44, 47, 56, 89, 100, 101, 104, 109
Information systems evaluation, 11, 12, 19, 36
Information Technology (IT), 7
Internet, 7, 37, 103, 109
Intranets, 109
Inventory control, 16
IS effectiveness, 17, 89
IS/IT, 5
IT/IS, 45, 54

L
Laboratory information systems, 1, 2, 15, 45, 47, 54, 58, 60, 62, 63, 65, 68, 74, 77, 78
Laboratory information systems development, 2, 59, 65, 80

M
Management considerations, 60, 69
Materials managers, 16
Medical pathology, 8, 15, 38, 39, 41, 43, 44, 57, 58, 73, 77, 88, 99
Middleware, 2, 65, 74
Mobilisation, 14

N
National Health Service (NHS), 11
Net present value (NPV), 24, 28

O
Open architecture systems, 2, 49
OpenLabs, 5, 46–48, 51, 108

M. Belkin et al., *Strategic ICT Planning in Pathology*,
Healthcare Delivery in the Information Age,
DOI 10.1007/978-1-4614-4478-7, © Springer Science+Business Media, LLC 2013

Printed in the United States
By Bookmasters